Your Personal Trainer is for all of you who are looking to
move your fitness and health to new levels,
using a time-efficient and accurate training approach that is *fun*,
results-oriented and proven.

To Jesus and my family . . . you bless me.

DSB

Contents

Preface

Committing to exercise is probably 70 percent of the battle toward achieving health, fitness, and performance benefits from a program of regular exercise. Nevertheless, many exercise enthusiasts and athletes are frustrated when they compare the time they spend exercising each week to the meager fitness improvements they have seen over an extended period of time. If that is your experience, you are not alone: millions of people worldwide echo these same "disappointment sentiments." My goal, working as your personal trainer, is to help you maximize fitness returns within the time frame to which you are currently dedicated.

Here are just a few of the problems you may be experiencing:

- You're not seeing the results you want despite investing hours per week working out.
- You're not quite sure how to progress your workouts to the next level.
- You'd like to add some variety to your workouts but don't know how, or even if it's a good idea.
- You're not losing weight (fat) or gaining muscle.
- Your performance in recreational or competitive sporting activities is not improving.
- You'd like to increase your aerobic endurance and get stronger, but it just isn't happening.
- You don't know how to easily measure and track fitness improvements so that you can evaluate the effectiveness of your training program.
- You don't know how to motivate yourself to keep exercising and stay committed.

Would you like a time-efficient formula that can move your workouts forward and help you attain higher levels of muscle strength, cardiovascular fitness, and flexibility? Would you like to have a sensible sport nutrition plan that you can follow easily and that fits into your active lifestyle? If you want to perform better in a sport or recreational activity; feel and look stronger; increase your muscle strength, size, and metabolism; have enough energy to last you an entire day; burn more fat and calories; and lose weight, then you've come to the right place.

If you continue to commit the time you're already investing in your workouts and follow my plan, you'll get results. *Your Personal Trainer* gives you the training advantage you need to create time-efficient workouts that guarantee training results.

Your Personal Trainer is a no-nonsense book, but it's fun and easy to read. This book will not point you toward fake-fat, electrical muscle stimulation units, and tanning beds. Instead you will find honest answers and practical solutions to all your health and fitness questions. You will also learn how to measure and improve your fitness, set realistic goals, and attain the results you've always wanted. *Your Personal Trainer* will show you how enjoyable exercise is when you're on the road to success. That's why you'll love this book and digest it from cover to cover!

Here's another plus. Think of this book as your chance to have your very own personal trainer at a fraction of the cost! Maybe you've always wanted to have your own personal trainer, but were not sure you wanted to make the investment. Or maybe you've worked with a trainer previously and understand firsthand what a difference it can make. A good personal trainer can update and change your workouts regularly, motivate you, give you up-to-date fitness and health information, and keep you on target so that you can accomplish your health and fitness goals. A trainer keeps your workouts time-efficient by keeping them focused and planned. *Your Personal Trainer* can help you with all of these things.

Your Personal Trainer is a compilation of information that I have learned over a period of 21 years. This is program design at its best and fitness training that works! I have used the information in this book with my clients and personally with great success over the years. This book presents advanced fitness information in an easy and fun format that you can start using today to improve your workouts. It will give your workouts a face-lift, keep the results coming, and keep you mentally fresh!

Here's the bottom line: if you've set aside time for your workouts, you should be able to accomplish your fitness goals. If you're frustrated and getting nowhere, this book is for you. *Your Personal Trainer* is based on a system that is time efficient, proven to work, and results oriented. It's what I call "smart training."

So, if you're a dedicated, self-motivated, and focused exerciser, or a personal trainer looking for new ideas and means to motivate your clients, give *Your Personal Trainer* a try. It puts practical, cutting-edge health and fitness information at your fingertips. The information, methods, and workout plans presented in this book have worked for me and my clients, as well as the thousands of fitness instructors and trainers I've trained, and continue to train, around the world.

Acknowledgments

A special thanks to the models who extended their warm energy, enthusiasm, and bodies to *Your Personal Trainer*. Candice Copeland, Cathy Dolan, Jeannie Eberts, John Kelly, Ilana Levin, Tom Nishikawa, and Robin Troutman—you are my friends and colleagues (and one my wife, too). Thanks for helping me to spread the fitness message.

A huge thank you to Snowcreek Athletic Club owner Tom Dempsey and club Manager Jarod Cogswell. Thanks for letting me use this wonderful facility to stage the photo shoot.

And, finally, to Human Kinetics Publishers (HKP), you are a talented team that knows "how to get it done"! A sincere thank you to Rainer Martens for seeing the vision, believing, and allowing it to happen; Martin Barnard (and Scott Wikgren) for your friendship and tireless efforts directed toward championing my involvement with several HKP projects; Rebecca Crist (and Marni Basic) who tirelessly and with a smile edited, formatted, and re-wrote *Your Personal Trainer* until it effectively communicated my ideas; Tom Roberts, you are the "camera-man"; and Marydell Forbes, you are the promotion guru workhorse. HKP you are a tireless team and relentless driving force behind every project. Thanks for your expertise and excellence!

PART I
Your Training Essentials

1 Self-Test Your Fitness Level

Your road to fitness and continued results starts from where you are, today. To create an exercise program that is goal and results oriented—or to jump-start workouts that are not getting you results—it's a good idea to know where you've been, where you are, and where you want to go.

In this chapter, you'll take stock of the first two items. To determine where you've been, you'll fill out a simple one-page medical history form. To determine where you are, you'll perform a series of self-assessment evaluations. Later, in chapter 2, you'll determine where you want to go by writing down your fitness goals.

This quick and easy three-step plan will help you identify your current fitness level and personal health status. This information will assist you in creating the most time-efficient and effective program, and will give you a starting point from which to compare your fitness improvements over time. Self-testing is not only a smart approach to optimizing training results, but also highly motivating.

WHERE YOU'VE BEEN

The most important first step, regardless of your actual fitness and perceived health status, is to fill out the one-page health and fitness medical history questionnaire on page 4. By thoroughly and honestly answering these questions, you will likely identify any questionable health areas. If you have any health concerns, or if the questionnaire "flags" an area you had never considered a risk, contact a qualified health care professional before beginning or continuing your exercise program. It is always prudent to receive your doctor's approval if you're just starting or changing an exercise program.

> **KEY POINT**
>
> It's in your interest to create a program that goes beyond physical activity and looks to broader personal health issues.

Even though you may be fit and active and think you are healthy, filling out a form like this will hold you accountable to your health history, may alert you to a few potential problem areas, and will highlight the importance of regular medical checkups (such as regular prostate or breast examinations) and maintaining a current relationship with your health care provider.

WHERE YOU ARE

Self-assessment can give you a realistic picture of the shape you're in and will help you establish sensible and attainable goals. Regular fitness checks also serve as a reference, or benchmark, to which you can compare your new training results over set periods of time. Because you'll be training smart, you will see improvements in cardiovascular fitness, muscular strength and endurance, and posture and flexibility. Your results will always compare to your starting point or most recent test, and not to those of other people (i.e., norms, percentiles, and rankings). These tests are quick and easy to do and serve as ongoing, powerful motivators that will keep you on track!

If you're not working out regularly and know you're out of shape, it is not necessary for you to test yourself. If you're deconditioned (consider yourself deconditioned if you work out sporadically or not at all), you may simply want to get your doctor's OK and get started on a program that builds gradually to higher levels of effort. After you have established a base level of fitness, you can then choose to test yourself. Using this approach, your body will be prepared for the physical effort of testing, and you'll be feeling more confident.

Self-assessment can help you find out what areas of your health and fitness program need improvement. It's painless and easy! Then, once you know where you stand, *Your Personal Trainer* shows you how to set goals, improve, and keep track of your results. Best of all, you can do the tests yourself. That means you don't need a partner, and if you prefer, no one else need know the outcome of your self-assessment tests.

Personal Health and Fitness Medical History Questionnaire

Name _____ Age _____ Date _____

Primary Health Care Provider _____

Provider's Contact Number _____

Other Health-Care Specialists:_____

Health history

1. Do you smoke?   Yes   No

   If you answered yes, how much do you smoke?_____

2. Has your doctor ever said your blood pressure was too high or too low?   Yes   No

3. Have you (or has a family member) been diagnosed with diabetes?   Yes   No

4. Do you have any known cardiovascular problems (heart disease,
   previous heart attack, atherosclerosis, abnormal ECG, etc.)?   Yes   No

   If you answered yes, please describe: _____

5. Has your doctor ever told you your cholesterol level was high?   Yes   No

6. Are you overweight?   Yes   No

   If you answered yes, how much are you overweight? _____

7. Do you have any injuries or orthopedic problems (bad back, bad knees,
   tendinitis, bursitis, etc.)?   Yes   No

   If you answered yes, please describe: _____

8. Are you taking any prescribed medications or dietary supplements?   Yes   No

   If you answered yes, please describe: _____

9. Are you pregnant or postpartum less than six weeks?   Yes   No

10. Date of last physical examination: _____

11. Do you have any other medical conditions or problems not previously mentioned?   Yes   No

    If you answered yes, please describe: _____

12. Describe your current exercise program: _____

_____

_____

13. List the goals of your program: _____

_____

_____

The remainder of this chapter describes several easy tests. The following four important areas of fitness are tested.

1. Body composition (how much fat, bone, and muscle you have)
2. Strength (how strong and fatigue resistant your muscles are)
3. Aerobic endurance (how strong your heart is)
4. Posture and flexibility (whether you can move easily with no major limitations or pain while maintaining good posture)

Some tests may not be appropriate for individuals with specific medical limitations or concerns. If you have any questions about the safety of a particular test, contact your doctor.

Over time, these tests will help you determine whether your program is working and help you recognize changes that are needed. Don't spend your time with a program that isn't working and will not help you accomplish your training goals. *Your Personal Trainer* will keep you progressing by giving you the programming options you need to customize your results and keep them coming. However, you have to be willing to change when change is warranted. Regular reevaluation (fitness checks) can help you make an objective decision.

KEY POINT

If you want to keep the results coming, you have to be willing to change when change is warranted!

BODY COMPOSITION

Why should you be worried about how much of you is fat, bone, and muscle? Having too much body fat has bigger implications than just cosmetics or a potentially negative impact on athletic performance. Too much fat is associated with an increased risk for heart disease, diabetes, some cancers, and many other health problems.

Although experts still argue about the ideal range of body fat, men should strive for between 12 and 18 percent and women for between 16 and 26 percent. Women naturally carry more fat than men because of the role women's bodies play in producing offspring. Competitive athletes generally have body fat measurements that fall below these percentages, depending on the sport they participate in and genetics.

If you choose to calculate your body fat, remember to focus on improvement from your starting point rather than concentrating on the actual percentage of fat and comparing it to norm standards. A long-term goal would be to progress in a positive direction relative to your starting point. Moreover, many "fat experts" argue that it may not be necessary to fall within these ranges to be healthy. However, optimal training results and health are probably more attainable if your body fat is within these ranges. Too much fat is bad for your health!

And yes, you can be too thin, although this is not the problem of most Americans. The last thing many dedicated exercisers need to do is lose body fat. Too little fat, especially in women, can lead to permanent bone loss and osteoporosis (bone-weakening disease), bone fractures, and irregular or missed menstrual periods.

The easiest and most useful way to measure fat and keep track of fat loss is by using fat calipers or a tape measure. Both methods are simple and inexpensive. Understanding the pros and cons of several methods used to document weight loss will help you grasp why calipers and tape measures are the right measurement tools for you to use.

Body Weight

Following daily body weight fluctuations can drive you to the point of insanity, if it hasn't already! Body weight (also called scale weight) is determined by using your bathroom scale. However, scale weight doesn't tell the whole story and can lead you astray. Your scale weight can go up or down a few pounds depending on how much, or how little, you have had to eat or drink before weighing or whether you have recently gone to the bathroom. Body weight fluctuations are also very common during a woman's normal menstrual cycle. Clothes can also increase your weight in varying amounts.

If you do weigh yourself, do it infrequently. To increase consistency with regard to comparing your most recent scale weight to a previous weight, weigh yourself at the same time (in the morning and before breakfast is a good time), use the same scale, and wear the same clothes or none at all.

Having said that, occasional weighing (about once every week or two) may help you spot an increase in weight. If you think it might be a fickle fluctuation (like water retention during a woman's menstrual cycle), check your body fat measurements with fat calipers or a tape measure (see resources in the appendix). If you've gained fat, an immediate reversal is called for. People who successfully keep large amounts of weight off say the secret to their success is to reverse small fat gains immediately.

Percent Body Fat

Percent body fat can be determined by using one of three popular methods: hydrostatic weighing, bioelectrical impedance (very high-tech but don't count on it being accurate), and skinfold measurements using fat calipers.

Hydrostatic Weighing

This method is often referred to as "underwater weighing" or the "dunk tank." Getting dunked involves sitting in a chair attached to a scale and being lowered into a tank of water. Sounds like a mess, doesn't it? There goes your perm or at least five dollars' worth of hair gel! This procedure can be fairly accurate, yet it requires a great deal of time, effort, expertise, and expense. This method serves as the "gold standard" to validate body fat percentage predictions using a fat caliper.

Bioelectrical Impedance

This procedure, often discussed in magazines and on TV, is based on the fact that electrical impulses sent through lean tissue (such as muscle) have greater conductivity than those sent through fat tissue. Don't let the electrodes attached to your body and the fancy computer printout fool you into thinking that this type of testing is quick, simple, and accurate. The results can vary wildly from test to test—by as much as 40 percent. Bioelectrical impedance is suspected of being inaccurate on many counts. In fact, no recognized industry standard for creating the formulas (they're programmed inside the computer) exists for these machines, and accurate results depend partially on the equation. In other words, the information the computer spits out is only as accurate as the formulas it is derived from.

The bioelectrical impedance test is less accurate than "dunking" and skinfold measurements because it tends to overestimate your body fat percentage if you are very lean and underestimate your body fat percentage if you have a lot of fat.

Skinfold Measurements

This is the most common fat test you'll run across. Skinfold calipers loosely resemble the pinchers on the face of a local pest. Fortunately, they do not feel the same. When you measure fat, you need to pull the fat away from the muscle firmly, but it is far from feeling like an ouch! A gauge on the calipers measures the thickness of the fat. (A skinfold is comprised of the two layers of skin you pinched plus the fat.) Most tests require three to seven different measurements to predict a body fat percentage.

Measuring Your Body Fat Using Skinfold Measurements

Performing skinfold measurements is easy. The fat caliper I recommend, Accu-Measure, requires only one simple measurement. A table developed by two very respected researchers, Dr. Andrew Jackson and Dr. Michael Pollock, and provided by the manufacturer allows you to cross-reference the single skinfold measure taken at your hip (the "love handle" area or iliac crest) with your age to find your percent body fat. Research has shown that this one-site measurement accurately represents the total amount of fat on the body. This piece of equipment moves you beyond the time-honored "pinch-an-inch," and gives you accurate results. Every fitness professional will tell you that body fat percentage is a very important index to monitor. With this procedure, testing your body fat couldn't be simpler or more cost effective, and it takes only seconds and can be done in the privacy of your home.

Follow these simple steps to use the skin caliper:

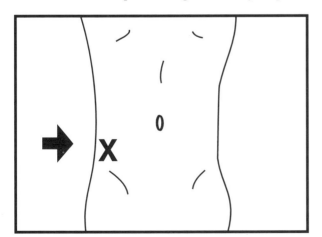

Figure 1.1 To measure your body fat using skin fold calipers, first find the iliac crest.

1. Locate the iliac crest, which is approximately one inch above the right hipbone (see figure 1.1).

2. While standing, firmly pinch the skinfold between your left thumb and fore finger (see figure 1.2). Place the jaws of the caliper over the skinfold while continuing to hold the skinfold with your left hand.

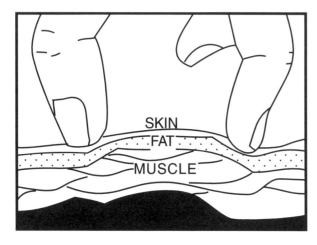 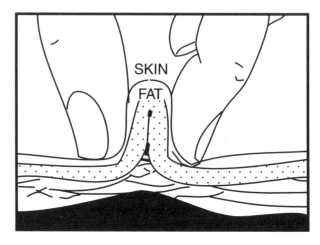

Figure 1.2 After locating the right spot, grab the skin and pinch.

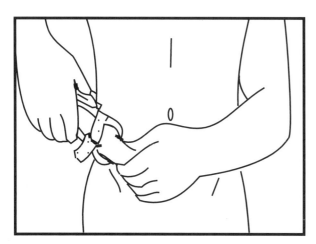

Figure 1.3 Use the calipers to measure the width of the pinched skin.

3. Press with your thumb where indicated on the caliper until you feel a slight click. The slide bar will automatically stop at the correct measurement (see figure 1.3). After reading your measurement, return the slide bar to the far right starting position. Repeat three times and use the average as your measurement. Use this average to determine your body fat percentage from table 1.1. Record your results in the body fat measurement sheet on page 10.

Be sure to take your measurement before exercise. Since blood travels to the skin to help cool your body during exercise, the skinfold measurement would be thicker right after a workout. This would make you test fatter—just what you don't need! Also, it's hard to grab that fat when your skin is slippery from sweat. If you follow these simple procedures your fat results will be very accurate.

Measuring Your Body Fat Using Tape Measurements

Measuring with a tape (a cloth measuring tape works the best) is another excellent and quick way to determine if you're losing fat. (It's a good idea to use both the skinfold calipers and tape measurements to monitor your body fat and body composition changes most effectively.)

Using the tape parallels the "How do your clothes fit?" line of thinking. If your pants are no longer snug, you know that you're losing inches. And if your tape measurements are shrinking, you know you're dropping fat!

Table 1.1 Skin Caliper Body Fat Percentage Chart

Males

Skinfold Measurements in Millimeters (mm)

Age in years	2–3	4–5	6–7	8–9	10–11	12–13	14–15	16–17	18–19	20–21	22–23	24–25	26–27	28–29	30–31	32–33	34–35
Up to 20	2.0	3.9	6.2	8.5	10.5	12.5	14.3	16.0	17.5	18.9	20.2	21.3	22.3	23.1	23.8	24.3	24.9
21–25	2.5	4.9	7.3	9.5	11.6	13.6	15.4	17.0	18.6	20.0	21.2	22.3	23.3	24.2	24.9	25.4	25.8
26–30	3.5	6.0	8.4	10.6	12.7	14.6	16.4	18.1	19.6	21.0	22.3	23.4	24.4	25.2	25.9	26.5	26.9
31–35	4.5	7.1	9.4	11.7	13.7	15.7	17.5	19.2	20.7	22.1	23.4	24.5	25.5	26.3	27.0	27.5	28.0
36–40	5.6	8.1	10.5	12.7	14.8	16.8	18.6	20.2	21.8	23.2	24.4	25.6	26.5	27.4	28.1	28.6	29.0
41–45	6.7	9.2	11.5	13.8	15.9	17.8	19.6	21.3	22.8	24.7	25.5	26.6	27.6	28.4	29.1	29.7	30.1
46–50	7.7	10.2	12.6	14.8	16.9	18.9	20.7	22.4	23.9	25.3	26.6	27.7	28.7	29.5	30.2	30.7	31.2
51–55	8.8	11.3	13.7	15.9	18.0	20.0	21.8	23.4	25.0	26.4	27.6	28.7	29.7	30.8	31.2	31.8	32.2
56 & up	9.9	12.4	14.7	17.0	19.0	21.0	22.8	24.5	26.0	27.4	28.7	29.8	30.8	31.6	32.3	32.9	33.3

Cross-reference your age with your measurement for your body fat percentage.

Females

Age in years	2–3	4–5	6–7	8–9	10–11	12–13	14–15	16–17	18–19	20–21	22–23	24–25	26–27	28–29	30–31	32–33	34–35
up to 20	11.3	13.5	15.7	17.7	19.7	21.5	23.2	24.8	26.3	27.7	29.0	30.2	31.3	32.3	33.1	33.9	34.6
21–25	11.9	14.2	16.3	18.4	20.3	22.1	23.8	25.5	27.0	28.4	29.6	30.8	31.9	32.9	33.8	34.5	35.2
26–30	12.5	14.8	16.9	19.0	20.9	22.7	24.5	26.1	27.6	29.0	30.3	31.5	32.5	33.5	34.4	35.2	35.8
31–35	13.2	15.4	17.6	19.6	21.5	23.4	25.1	26.7	28.2	29.6	30.9	32.1	33.2	34.1	35.0	35.8	36.4
36–40	13.8	16.0	18.2	20.2	22.2	24.0	25.7	27.3	28.8	30.2	31.5	32.7	33.8	34.8	35.6	36.4	37.0
41–45	14.4	16.7	18.8	20.8	22.8	24.6	26.3	27.9	29.4	30.8	32.1	33.3	34.4	35.4	36.3	37.0	37.7
46–50	15.0	17.3	19.4	21.5	23.4	25.2	26.9	28.6	30.1	31.5	32.8	34.0	35.0	36.0	36.9	37.6	38.3
51–55	15.6	17.9	20.0	22.1	24.0	25.9	27.6	29.2	30.7	32.1	33.4	34.6	35.6	36.6	37.5	38.3	38.9
56 & up	16.3	18.5	20.7	22.7	24.6	26.5	28.2	29.8	31.3	32.7	34.0	35.2	36.3	37.2	38.1	38.9	39.5

Body Fat Measurement Sheet (Using Skinfold Calipers)

Name _____ Age _____ Start date _____

Measurement date								
Scale weight (optional)								
Body fat (measured in millimeters)*								
Measurement site (iliac crest or "love handle")								
Percentage body fat								

* Simply read your Accu-Measure caliper, which is calibrated in millimeters, and record the number. Cross reference your age with your measurement in table 1.1 to find your body fat percentage.

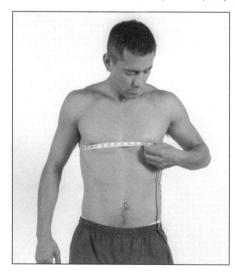

Keep the body part being measured relaxed. While there are many possible measurement locations, the following five are most important and don't require a helper. Record your results for each measurement in the Tape Measurement Record-Keeping Sheet on page 12.

1. Chest. Take this measurement at nipple level. Run the tape from behind you toward the front (see figure 1.4).

Figure 1.4 Tape measurement for chest.

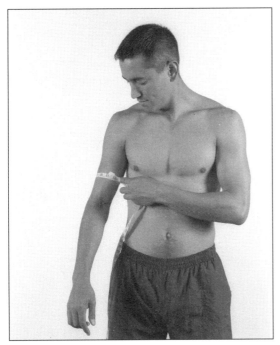

Figure 1.5   Tape measurement for upper arm.

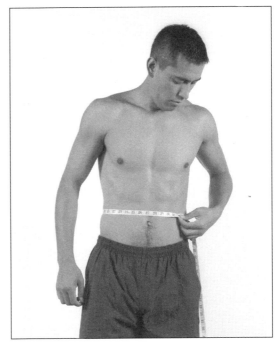

Figure 1.6   Tape measurement for waist.

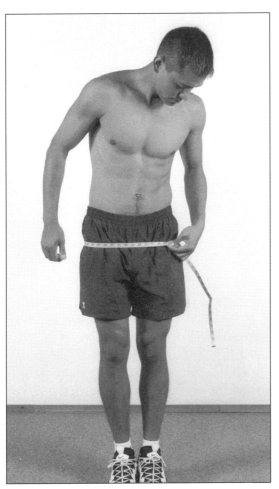

2. Upper Arm. Take this measurement around the largest part of the upper arm. The arm being measured is hanging downward and relaxed (see figure 1.5). You can do this by yourself if you assist your hands by using a piece of sticky tape to attach one end of the cloth tape to your arm. (If you don't want to use tape, you'll have to hold one end of the measurement tape in place with your nose!)

3. Waist. Take this measurement at the narrowest point (believe it or not, you have a narrowest point!) of your waist. Run the tape from behind you toward the front (see figure 1.6).

4. Hips. Take this measurement standing, with your feet together (see figure 1.7). Run the tape from behind you and around the "greatest protrusion" of the buttocks (where your buttocks stick out the farthest).

Figure 1.7   Tape measurement for hips.

Tape Measurements Record-Keeping Sheet

Name _____   Age _____   Start Date _____

Tape measure site locations (measured in inches with a cloth tape):

Measurement Date:						
Chest:						
Upper arm:						
Waist:						
Hips:						
Thigh:						

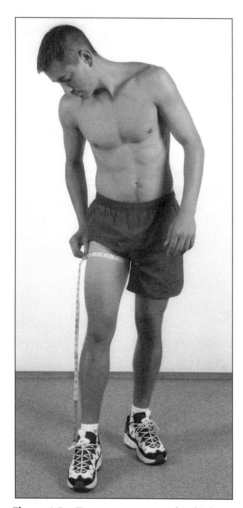

Figure 1.8   Tape measurement for thigh.

5. Thigh. Take this measurement around the largest part of the upper leg, which is usually just below the buttocks or gluteal fold (see figure 1.8).

STRENGTH TESTING

Muscular endurance and muscular strength fall under the strength testing heading. Muscular strength can be characterized as the ability of your muscles to produce high levels of force for short time periods (i.e., 30 to 90 seconds). Muscular endurance is defined as the muscles' ability to fight off fatigue for longer periods of time. Both are important to improved athletic performance, effective and safe daily movement, and good posture.

Testing Muscular Endurance

Has anyone ever asked you how "endurant" your muscles are? Probably not, but don't let this lead you to believe that it's not important. The ability to sustain muscle contraction (or exerting force without fatiguing quickly) over longer time periods can help you, for example, maintain proper skill execution (skill levels decrease when fatigue sets in) and correct posture (maintaining proper posture throughout the day requires muscular endurance).

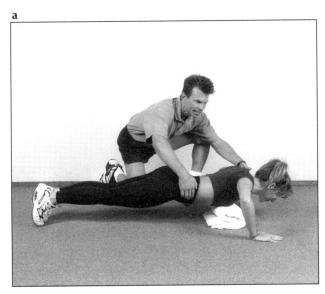
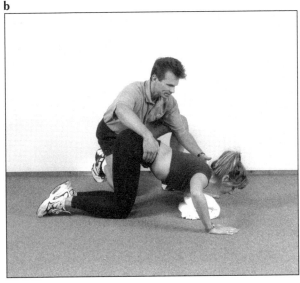

Figure 1.9   *(a)* A standard push-up should be performed with the back straight, the hands about shoulder-width apart, and the head is neither up or down. Only your feet and hands contact the floor in the starting position. *(b)* For the modified bent-knee version the only difference is that your knees should rest on the floor, bent at a 90° angle with the ankles hip width apart.

Nonsexist Push-Up Test

Implying that women should perform modified or bent-leg push-ups and men standard, straight-body push-ups is sexist. Period. Whether or not you perform a bent-knee or straight-body push-up depends on upper body strength. Period. If you don't think you can do at least 13 (anything below this number and you're measuring muscle strength!) straight-body or standard push-ups, then opt to use the modified, bent-knee version. See figure 1.9a–b.

If you choose to do the push-up test, men and women may perform either the bent-knee or standard (straight-body) push-up. The goal of the push-up test is to perform the most push-ups you can. This test measures the endurance and, to some degree, the strength of your chest, shoulder, and arm muscles.

A light aerobic warm-up and gentle stretching of the upper body should precede this test. After you choose the style of push-up, lower your chest toward the floor until it touches a rolled-up towel (about three inches thick) and return to a straight-arm position. Perform the push-up with control, using one second up and one second down as a guide. If you have a metronome, set it at 60 beats per minute. If you don't have a metronome, the testing won't be as exact when you try to replicate the test for future comparisons, but you can simply count, for example, "one thousand one" and repeat this count when you reverse direction.

Lower your entire body and keep your back from sagging. You must push up to a straight-arm position on each repetition to have it count toward your test score. The test score is the total number of push-ups you complete. When you can't return to the straight-arm start position or maintain an even rhythm, the test is over. Record the number of push-ups you did on the Muscular Endurance Testing Sheet on page 14 and retest four to six weeks later.

You may want to calculate personal percentage improvement after your first retest, and thereafter (see chapter 15). Or, you can simply note how many more push-ups you're able to do after each retest.

Muscular Endurance Testing Sheet (Push-Ups)

Name _____   Age _____   Start date _____

Measurement date										
Number of push-ups completed										
Bent-knee push-up										
Straight-body or standard push-up										

Curl-Up Crunch Test

The "old" sit-up tests were used to measure a full sit-up. Generally, your feet were held, and with reckless abandon you did as many sit-ups as you could in 60 seconds. However, the sit-up is not a good measure of abdominal strength/endurance because it uses hip flexor muscles and puts unnecessary stress on your back and spine.

The curl-up crunch test has no time limit and teaches good exercise technique. However, if you have a history of back pain, check with your doctor or don't do this test. A light aerobic warm-up and gentle stretching should precede this test.

The goal of the curl-up test is to count the maximum number of abdominal crunches you can do before reaching muscular failure (can't do another one with good form). It is a good indicator of abdominal muscle endurance, or lack of it.

To set up the test, lie on your back with your arms at your sides, palms facing down. Without lifting your head or shoulders, reach with your fingers toward your feet and press your shoulders away from your ears. Place horizontal pieces of tape at the farthest points the fingers touched. Place two more pieces of tape two and a half inches beyond these marks (see figure 1.10a–b).

To perform the test, lie on your back with your palms facing down and your fingertips resting on the edges of the top pieces of tape closest to your shoulders. Make sure your shoulders are pressed down and away from your ears. Bend your knees by placing them a comfortable distance away from your buttocks and keep your feet flat on the floor. Now, focus on drawing your ribs down toward your hips. As a consequence, your head, shoulders, and torso will lift.

a

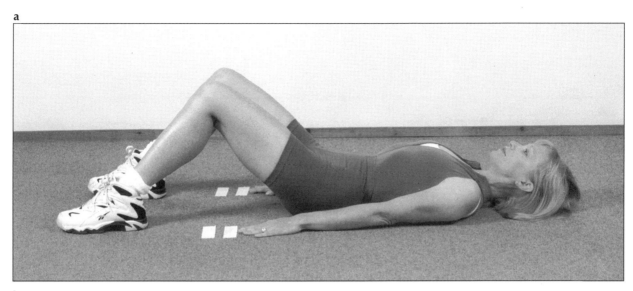

b

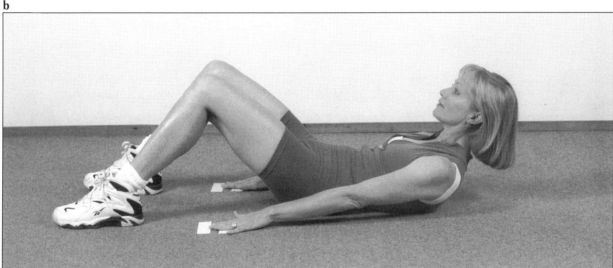

Figure 1.10   *(a)* Start position of Curl-up Crunch test.   *(b)* End position of Curl-up Crunch test.

Slide your fingertips along the floor until they touch the top edges of the lower tape markings. Return to the starting position and keep performing the crunch (with control, about two seconds up and two seconds down) until you can't do any more, can no longer touch the bottom pieces of tape, or cannot maintain the rhythm you started the test with (two seconds up, two seconds down). Remember, the fingertips of both hands must touch the bottom tape markings on either side of your body to count as a repetition. Touching both pieces of tape also keeps you from moving only one side of your body. The curl-up crunch test score is the number of controlled touches you make on the bottom tape marks.

Record your total number of repetitions on the Muscular Endurance Testing Sheet for Crunches on page 16 so that you can compare your performance to future efforts. You may want to calculate personal percentage improvement after your first retest, and thereafter. Or, you can simply note how many more curl-ups you're able to do after each retest.

Muscular Endurance Testing Sheet (Crunches)

Name _____ Age _____ Start date _____

Measurement date										
Number of curl-ups completed										
Modified curl-up or crunch										

Testing Muscular Strength

Everybody wants to know how strong they are. After as little as four to six weeks of smart training you'll see dramatic improvements in your strength, regardless of where you started. So naturally you'll want to measure how well you're doing. Be careful you don't hurt yourself! Going about it incorrectly will sabotage the best of intentions by making you unable to exercise regularly!

Perform this test only after training with heavier resistance, for example 8 to 12 repetitions performed to fatigue, for at least four to six weeks.

Rest time between any repeat attempts should be about two to five minutes to make sure your muscles are recovered and ready to go again.

During the repetitions, maintain proper breathing technique. Exhale as you move the weight away from the starting position and inhale as you slowly bring it back. Never hold your breath. Breath holding can significantly increase pressure in the chest, raising blood pressure and heart rate to unnecessarily high and potentially dangerous levels.

A strength test requires an aerobic warm-up. You can also include a couple of lightweight warm-up sets and gentle stretching prior to the test. A proper warm-up, along with the help of a spotter, will enable you to perform this test in the safest manner. It's a good idea to have a personal trainer or skilled workout partner supervise and spot the test for maximum safety. A spotter should be there to help you in case you are unable to complete the number of repetitions you had planned.

Maintain control through each lifting movement. Use two seconds up and two seconds down. If you have a metronome, set it at 30 beats per minute (two seconds up and two seconds down). If you don't have a metronome, the testing won't be as exact when you try to replicate the test for future comparisons, but you can simply count, for example, "one thousand one, one thousand two" and repeat this count when you reverse direction.

After the test, record the amount of weight lifted and the number of reps completed on page 18. Any repetition in which the spotter does any of the work should not be included in the final count.

Muscular Strength Test:
8- to 12-Repetition Maximum (RM) to Fatigue

What's great about the 8- to 12-RM test is that you can use any common exercise(s) and equipment that you're currently using. (An RM represents the most amount of weight you can lift with good form. A 1-RM represents the most amount of weight you can lift once, whereas a 10-RM is the most amount of weight you can lift ten times without losing form.) A light aerobic warm-up and gentle stretching of the upper body should precede this test.

After warming up, choose any exercise(s) and use enough resistance to cause your muscles to fatigue between 8 and 12 reps. (If you do more than 12 reps, add more weight.) Perform the exercise in a controlled manner—for example, two seconds up and two seconds down. If you cannot finish a rep (be sure you're spotted) or can no longer maintain a smooth rhythm, the test is over. Record the number of reps and weight lifted on the 8- to 12-Repetition Maximum Test Sheet on page 18.

If you're using elastic resistance, count the number of times the tubing is wrapped around your hand (this makes it harder) or note how far you're standing from its attachment point in the door (the farther you are from the attachment, the harder it is).

Retest about four to six weeks later using the same weight and procedures. You'll probably be able to do more repetitions. This indicates an increase in strength. By the way, if you're getting stronger, your muscles are also becoming more endurant, or fatigue resistance. As you get stronger, you can do more repetitions for any given amount of weight you could lift before you earned your newly won gains in strength. At some point, for example, after several retests, increase your resistance so that you fatigue between 8 and 12 reps again. Retest using this new resistance. Being able to do more reps and progressively increasing resistance are good indicators that your strength training program is working.

CARDIOVASCULAR ENDURANCE TESTING

How strong is your heart? You may have heard a friend or someone at the gym talking about a "submax O_2 test," and you've probably thought, "What in the world is that?" "Submax" is short for "submaximal" and tells you that you're working at a level of effort below "all-out." This usually equates to about 70 to 85 percent of your maximal heart rate, or a level of effort (referred to as rating of perceived exertion or RPE) that is from 3 to 7 ("moderate" to "hard"). Submax tests give you an idea of how strong your heart is and how well it can pump oxygen to your muscles. The more fit your heart is, the more calories you can burn, and you'll have more energy! An all-out maximal test should only be done in a medically supervised setting.

A comparison of your submax test results can help you evaluate whether your aerobic training is effective and motivate you toward new goals. It is an objective measure that will show whether you're on-track!

Submax tests should be preceded by an easy warm-up of at least three to five minutes and followed with a gradual cool-down of three to five minutes and stretching.

Muscular Strength Testing Sheet (8-12 Repetition Maximum)

Name _____ Age _____ Start date _____

Measurement date					
Exercise	Reps/weight	Reps/weight	Reps/weight	Reps/weight	Reps/weight

One-Mile Walk/Run Test

The one-mile walk/run test is the simplest way to submaximally test your aerobic fitness. This test requires a watch that measures seconds and a measured one-mile walking/running route. (If this distance seems intimidating or too long, create a course of any length and follow the procedures.)

Before you walk, walk and run, or run the course, warm up for three to five minutes. Then, cover the route as fast as you can and record the time it takes you. A trained speed walker may finish in 8 to 9 minutes (a speed of 7.5 to 6.7 mph), while a fast runner may complete the course in 6 minutes (a speed of 10 mph). If you're out of shape, you might take as long as 30 minutes (a speed of 2.0 mph) plus. No matter! Simply note how much time it took you to complete your mile course.

Take your pulse for 10 seconds immediately upon completing the course. This is called your exercise heart rate (EHR). Measure your heart rate at the radial pulse near your thumb and wrist, or use a heart rate monitor. Multiply this number by 6 to get your heart rate count for one minute. For example, if you counted 20 beats in 10 seconds, 20 multiplied by 6 equals 120 beats per minute.

One minute after you stopped exercising, take your pulse again for another 10-second count. This second pulse measure is called the recovery heart rate (RyHR).

Record this information on the Aerobic Test Evaluation Sheet (page 20).

When you retest four to six weeks later, you'll be pleased by how much faster you can complete this same course, and you may have progressed from a walk to a run. In addition, your exercise heart rate and recovery heart rate will be lower (meaning the test is easier and you recover from the effort more quickly) when compared to your previous test. Your faster speed, lower exercising heart rate (taken right after you finish the mile), and lower recovery heart rate (taken one minute after you finish) are excellent indicators that your program is working.

Step Test

Typically you'll see this test performed with a 12-inch step. However, for some people a 12-inch step is too high. It may cause them to reach a maximal or high heart rate quickly, or the height of the step could stress their knees. You can test using any step height; just be sure to retest using the same height. (The 12-inch height is used most often so you can use the associated norms and/or percentile ranking to rate your performances.) If you like numbers and statistics, just calculate your personal percentage improvement (see chapter 15) when you retest and you won't have to step on such a high height.

During the test, try to step at a steady cadence that you can replicate from test to test. For example, count "up" (right foot), "up" (left foot), "down" (right foot), "down" (left foot) and take about one second for each "up," "up," "down," "down," or a total of four seconds. If you have a metronome, set it for 60 beats per minute and step with the same "up, up, down, down" rhythm.

Use the first step of a stairway or a small, stable platform to step on. The platform should be no higher than 12 inches. Any height that is less, works. Step up and down on the step or platform for three minutes.

a

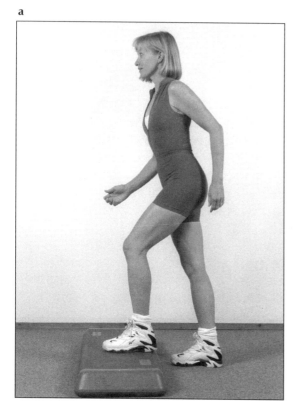

b

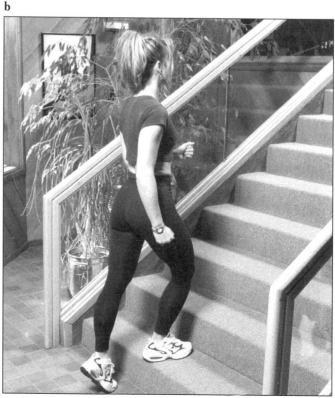

Figure 1.11 *(a)* Performing the step test on a 4-inch step platform. *(b)* Performing the step test on a stair step.

Aerobic Test Evaluation Sheet

(Use this form for the one mile walk/run and steps tests.)

Name _____ **Age** _____ **Start date** _____

Measurement date									

Record your one-minute exercise heart rate (EHR) and recovery heart rate (RyHR) in each box. Find HR by taking a 10-second heart rate count and multiplying the 10-second count by 6.

One-Mile Walk, Walk and Run, or Run

EHR Example:120									
RyHR: Example:80									

Step Test

EHr: Example:135									
RyHR: Example:85									

Your exercise heart rate is determined by taking your pulse for 10 seconds immediately upon completing the three-minute stepping duration. Measure your heart rate at the radial pulse near your thumb and wrist, or use a heart rate monitor. Multiply this number by 6 to get your heart rate count for one minute. For example, if you counted 20 beats in 10 seconds, 20 multiplied by 6 equals 120 beats per minute.

One minute after you stopped exercising, take your pulse again for another 10-second count to determine your recovery heart rate (RyHR).

Record this information on the Aerobic Test Evaluation Sheet (page 20).

If you follow this same procedure each time you test, you can get a reliable result that can be used to evaluate changes in your aerobic fitness. Be sure to use the same step height and procedure for each retest.

When you retest four to six weeks later, you'll be pleased by how much easier it feels to complete the three-minute stepping duration. In addition, your exercise heart rate and recovery heart rate will be lower (meaning your aerobic fitness has improved and you recover from the effort more quickly) compared to your previous test. Your lower exercising heart rate (taken right after you finish stepping) and lower recovery heart rate (taken one minute after you finish) are excellent indicators that your program is working.

POSTURE AND FLEXIBILITY

For most people "good" posture does not occur naturally but happens when you gain an awareness of how your posture compares to "good" posture. Is your head forward and chin jutted toward the ceiling? Is your upper back rounded, and do you walk with that "hunched-over" look? Poor posture and chronic misalignment of your neck, shoulders, and hips can lead to pain during rest or play and places a lot of stress on your joints, ligaments, and muscles.

Poor posture can be changed consciously with strengthening, stretching, and "posture checks" throughout the day. (Are you slouching in your chair?) Good body alignment is important not only for improving performance, but also to prevent pain, discomfort, and injury.

Flexibility (affected by poor posture) is simply defined as how far and how easily you can move your joints. This is a measure of how tight your muscles are. Unrestricted and easy movement are important for safety reasons, efficient exercise, and participating effectively in daily tasks.

Posture Assessment

All posture and flexibility assessment tests should include a three- to five-minute warm-up and gentle stretching prior to the tests. This will help you avoid injury and allow you to perform the test better. All of the tests should be performed with control. Never force your body to a point of pain or extreme discomfort.

This section will help you identify your posture as "good" or "needs improvement" and will also show you how to create correct posture. When you screen yourself for posture, wear minimal clothing (like a bathing suit), no

Posture Assessment Check Sheet

Head and Upper Back

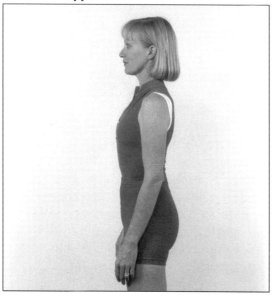

Good head posture: Head aligned over shoulders

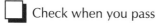 Check when you pass

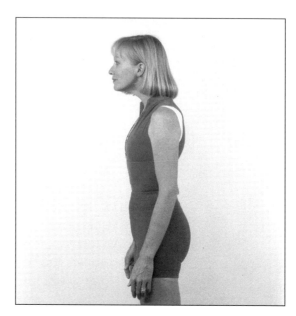

Needs some work: Chin jutted forward

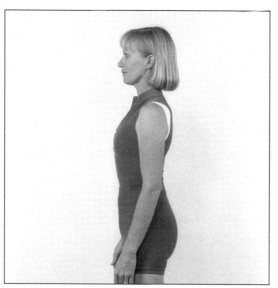

Good upper back posture: Shoulders pulled slightly back

Check when you pass

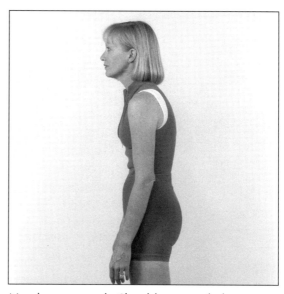

Needs some work: Shoulders rounded

Solution:

A forward head position usually occurs because of weak upper back muscles and tight shoulder and chest muscles and is a compensatory posture resulting from the resultant hunched-over position of the upper back. This misaligned head position can be corrected by reversing this rounded-shoulder and hunched-back posture. Simply stretch the front of your shoulders and chest muscles and strengthen your upper back.

Posture Assessment Check Sheet *continued*

Low Back and Abdominals

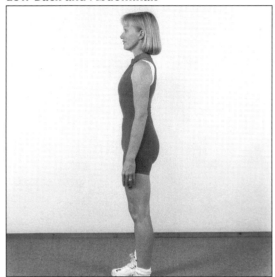

Good low back posture: Head, shoulders, hips, and ankles are aligned. A natural curve is present in the low back and neck area

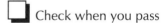 Check when you pass

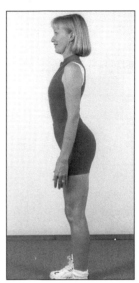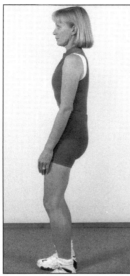

Needs some work: Arched back or flat back

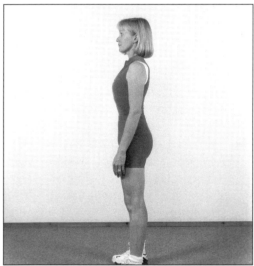

Good abdominal posture: Stomach does not stick out beyond the chest

Check when you pass

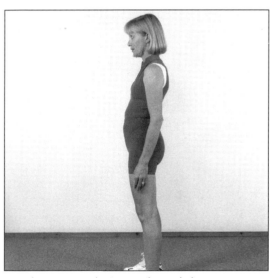

Needs some work: Stomach or abdomen is protruding

Solution:

If your back is excessively arched, stretch your hip flexors (front of the hip). Although tight back muscles may cause your low back to be arched and your abdomen to protrude, this usually is not the case. Because most people sit in cars and office chairs with poor posture (rounded low back and upper back), the lower back muscles are usually overstretched and weak. Consequently, it is usually not necessary to stretch these muscles. Instead, strengthen your abdominal muscles to correct a protruding abdomen and an arched back, and stretch the hip flexors.

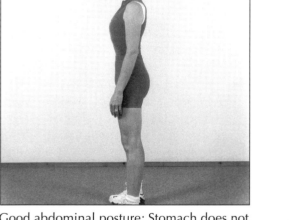

shoes, and do the screening in front of a mirror. Assume a relaxed, normal posture. Don't try to correct poor posture during the test.

Repeat these tests every four to six weeks to monitor your progress. After you successfully pass these tests, be sure to continue the stretching and strengthening exercises that helped you improve your posture and reach new levels of flexibility.

Don't forget to strengthen your back muscles, too. Strong back muscles are important for a healthy back!

If your back is more flat than arched, it's probably a good idea to stretch the back of your upper legs (hamstrings).

If you have pain or discomfort, or questions regarding the right approach to improving your spinal posture and back health, contact your doctor. If you notice any of the following postural deviations while assessing your body posture in the mirror, you may want to discuss these with your doctor.

- Hyperextended knees or knees that "push back"
- Excessively high arches
- A second toe that is longer than the big toe (Morton's foot)
- Uneven shoulders or hips
- Bowed legs (knees are apart when ankles touch)
- Knock-knees(knees touch when feet are apart)
- Sideways curvature of the spine (scoliosis)
- Ankles that are excessively rolled in (overpronation) or excessively rolled out (oversupination)

WHAT DO YOU DO WITH YOUR TEST RESULTS?

After you conduct the test outlined on the following pages, write down your results on the testing sheets. What you shouldn't do is file them so well you forget where you've stored them. Instead, use your results and *Your Personal Trainer* to create your plan of attack. Chapter 2 will help you set your plan of action and organize your workouts. Chapter 3 will help you choose the right equipment. Chapters 4, 5, 6, and 7 will show you the best programs and techniques for stretching your body, training your heart, and strengthening your muscles. Chapter 8 introduces variety and cross-training, whereas chapter 9 emphasizes the importance of balancing effort and recovery. Eating for your health and exercise performance makes up chapter 10. Chapters 11, 12, 13, and 14 give you specialized programs to follow and the tools to create your own customized workout plan. Chapter 15 brings you full circle and discusses the importance of tracking your progress with reassessment tests, calculating percent improvement, and keeping your fitness progressing to the next level.

Parts of this chapter were adapted or reprinted with permission from FitnessTrakker, a record-keeping and motivational system created and written by Derrick Pedranti and Douglas Brooks, 1997.

Flexibility Check Sheet

* See chapter 4 for instructions on performing these stretches and chapter 7 for strengthening exercises that can help improve your posture.

Shoulders (outward rotation)

Instructions: Raise your hand behind your head and down toward the opposite shoulder blade

Goal: To touch the top of the opposite shoulder blade

Stretches:

- shoulder press backward overhead or down
- triceps stretch overhead

☐ Check when you pass

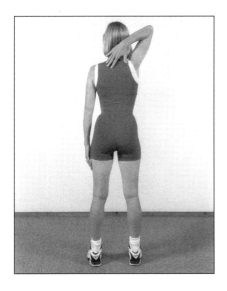

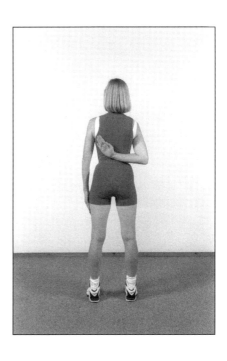

Shoulders (inward rotation)

Insruction: Turn your palm facing behind you and place it in the low back.Raise your hand toward the opposite shoulder blade

Goal: To touch the bottom of the opposite shoulder blade

Stretches:

- Shoulder pull-back: clasp your hands together behind your body and lift your arms

☐ Check when you pass

Low back

Instructions: Lie on your back and pull both knees toward your chest by grasping the back of your thighs with your hands

Goal: To have the upper thighs touch the chest

Stretches:

- single- or double-knee stretches to the chest
- cat back

☐ Check when you pass

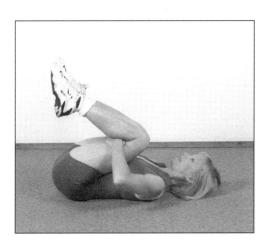

Flexibility Check Sheet *continued*

Front of hips (hip flexors)

Instruction: Lie on your back with one leg straight and hug the other leg to your chest by grasping the back of your thigh with your hands

Goal: To have the upper thigh of the bent leg touch the chest while the back of the lower leg of the straight leg remains in contact with the floor; the knee of the straight leg must not bend

Stretches:

- kneeling or standing hip flexor stretches

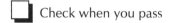 Check when you pass

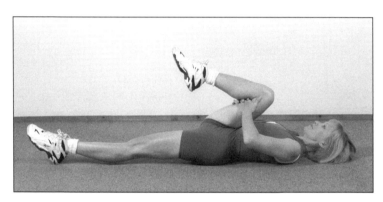

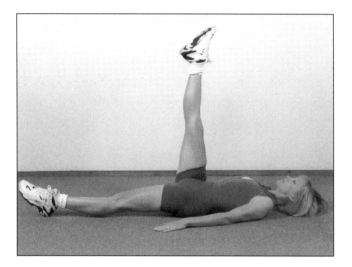

Back of the thighs (hamstrings)

Instructions: Lie on your back with both legs flat on the floor; then lift one leg upward

Goal: To lift one leg to a vertical position without bending either knee

Stretches:

- standing or lying hamstring stretches

☐ Check when you pass

Front of thighs (quadriceps)

Instructions: Lie on your stomach with your knees together; keep one leg straight and pull the heel toward the buttocks by grasping the top of your foot (shoe laces) with the hand that's on the same side of the leg you're stretching

Goal: To draw the heel toward and to easily touch the heel to the buttocks

Stretches:

- standing or lying quadriceps stretches

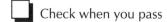 Check when you pass

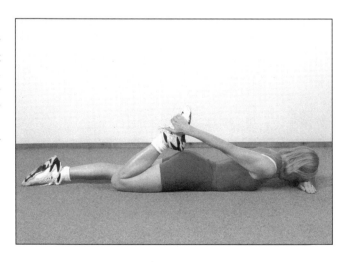

Flexibility Check Sheet *continued*

Calves and ankles

Instructions: Sit on the floor with an upright posture or lean back slightly with your arms supported behind you; position your legs straight out in front of you; draw your toe toward your shin

Goal: To easily move your toes toward your shin so that they are past perpendicular to the floor/ceiling

Stretches:

- standing wall press
- seated calf stretch

☐ Check when you pass

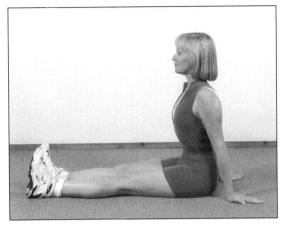

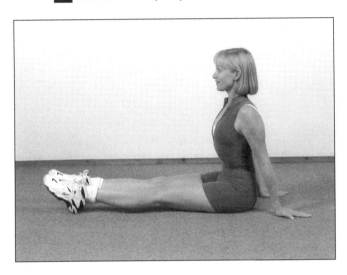

Shins and ankles

Instructions: Sit on the floor with an upright posture or lean back slightly with your arms supported behind you; position your legs straight out in front of you; point your toes away from you toward the floor

Goal: To move your toes from an orientation toward the ceiling (90 degrees) to a position of 45 degrees (bottom of foot is 3–4 inches from floor)

Stretches:

- Shin or tibialis stretches

☐ Check when you pass

Quick Index:

2 Set a Planned Course of Action

It has been said, if you keep doing what you have always done, you will get what you have always gotten. Your workout program cannot proceed according to a plan if you have no plan, nor can you expect great results without a road map to guide you.

The questions "How much exercise is enough?" and "What type of exercise is best for developing and maintaining fitness?" are asked by anyone who's serious about a training program. The question that usually follows is, "How can I devise a training program that gets me the results I want in a time-effective way?" These are good "cut-to-the-chase" questions, and you'll find the answers in chapters 4 through 15. But, before digesting the information found in these chapters, take a few minutes to set realistic goals and organize your training, and you'll find the information in *Your Personal Trainer* more useful.

Too often, individuals set goals and never revisit them. Setting and reevaluating personal goals keeps you accountable; keeps your training program, mind, and body fresh; and keeps the results coming in. Before you set your goals, you need to ask yourself, am I training for health or fitness? And, am I willing to reevaluate and change directions when the evidence warrants it?

ARE YOU TRAINING FOR HEALTH OR FITNESS?

In July 1993, the American College of Sports Medicine (ACSM) and the Centers for Disease Control (CDC), in cooperation with the President's Council on Physical Fitness and Sports, released a statement announcing that a persuasive body of scientific evidence indicates that regular, moderate-intensity physical activity offers substantial health benefits to the public.

The 1993 recommendations state that every adult should accumulate 30 minutes or more of moderate-intensity physical activity over the course of most days of the week. Additionally, performing a series of short bouts of exercise of moderate intensity, lasting from about 8 to 10 minutes with total duration being at least 30 minutes per day, will also provide significant and similar health benefits when compared to exercising for 30 minutes all at one time. In other words, the total amount of activity is the key, not whether it is performed continuously. That is good news for someone who finds 30 minutes of continuous activity, of any kind, rather daunting.

The statement further recommends incorporating activity into daily routines. This is time-efficient and nonintimidating. Examples of effective activity include walking stairs instead of riding elevators, gardening, raking leaves, shoveling snow, dancing, vigorously cleaning house, and strolling. Planned exercise or recreational activity such as an aerobics class, hiking, biking, tennis, swimming, or strength training may also be used.

It is now clear that lower levels of physical activity may reduce the risk for certain chronic degenerative diseases. This is not an issue of right and wrong, or easy versus moderate or vigorous exercise, but an issue of personal knowledge, appropriateness, and encouraging a majority of the population to exercise effectively.

Physical fitness is made up of the right combination of amount and intensity of cardiovascular fitness, muscular strength and endurance, and flexibility training. It is also important to monitor body composition (how much fat you have). Fitness is often stiffly defined as the ability to perform moderate to vigorous levels of physical activity without undue fatigue. That statement probably doesn't mean a whole lot to you. More important, fitness training should encompass the capability and personal desire to maintain this activity level throughout life while experiencing a consistent level of enjoyment—you should like what you're doing!

KEY POINT

Many of you reading this book will be looking to move beyond moderate physical activity and toward optimizing your health, fitness, and performance training returns. If this is true, let your goals reflect this direction.

DESCRIBE AND RECORD YOUR GOALS

Setting goals and record keeping are important because the adaptive response to training (becoming more fit from working harder) is complex and individual. In other words, individuals will most likely respond differently to exactly the same program. Because of this, it is important to update your goals and record your progress or lack thereof so that appropriate changes can be made to create improvement or continued gains in your fitness.

If this concept of developing goals is to be useful, you must (1) commit them to paper, (2) be specific, (3) set realistic goals, and (4) read and reevaluate your goals regularly.

Writing Goals

Develop both short-term, mid-term, and long-term goals. Short-term goals should be attainable in about four to eight weeks and mid-term goals from eight weeks to six months. Attainment of success in shorter time periods will keep your desire pumped and your commitment to exercise high. Long-term goals can be reached any time after six months, and might not be attained for a year or longer.

Identifying Your Fitness Goals

Several fitness and health goals that you'd like to achieve have probably already popped into your head. Use the ideas in the Goal-Setting Checklist to stimulate further thought. Then, add any new goal ideas to the personal goals you've already thought of but maybe haven't written down on the Fitness Goal Tracking Form (pages 32-33). Using the Goal-Setting Checklist will help ensure that your goal list covers all of your health and fitness needs. A good personal trainer puts this kind of thought process to work in designing the best program for a client, and that's just what *Your Personal Trainer* does for you!

Goal-Setting Checklist

When you can express what you want to accomplish on paper, it programs your mind and body to achieve that goal. Start with a few targets (goals). You can't hit a target unless you have at least one! Setting goals help you understand what motivates you to work out.

1. Identify why you are exercising. Looking, performing, and feeling better are good long-term goals, but don't forget about short-term, specific goals. A good short-term goal might be to strength train three days per week. This is realistic and achievable and will serve to motivate you until you reach your loftier or more ambiguous goals.

2. What motivates you to exercise? Ask yourself, and write it down. It will help you develop goals that work for you.

3. Orient yourself to a variety of activities. This will help you avoid boredom and overuse injuries and find activities you enjoy.

4. Consider your level of enjoyment when exercising. If you like what you're doing, you'll be more likely to incorporate fitness into a permanent lifestyle change.

5. Commit to exercising regularly. Set minimum (life is hectic) and optimum (life is under control) training schedules. If you do this, you're more likely to stay active and get results (which by itself is motivating). Repeat this phrase: exercise is a year-round habit, like personal hygiene. It is not a part-time hobby. Plus, health and fitness are easier to maintain than regain!

6. Keep your workouts at reasonable lengths. Is this a schedule you can realistically commit to for a lifetime and still maintain other important responsibilities? Make sure the number of days you work out and the duration of your workouts are in line with what you want to accomplish. Be realistic! While you can attain substantial health and fitness benefits from three workouts per week, you won't be competitive on a world-class level!

7. Identify the "big picture." Through your commitment to consistent workouts and other positive lifestyle changes, keep in mind the ultimate goal of improving your quality of life.

8. Write specific goals. Be as specific as possible in detailing the goal and how you are going to attain it. Fitness goals can be performance or health related, or as simple as lifting more weight, losing fat, and exercising regularly. Then put your plan into action. Use the information in *Your Personal Trainer* to ensure a balanced approach. Furthermore, take the steps necessary to make it happen (schedule it) and adjust your plans when necessary.

9. Schedule and organize your day. People who exercise in the morning are more likely to stick with their programs. Regardless, somehow schedule exercise into your day so that it gets done. View it as an important appointment you would not dare miss and selfishly protect this sacred time. Written plans are more likely to be accomplished than good intentions, so don't just think it, ink it!

10. Spend a reasonable effort exercising. If you're going to spend the time exercising, why not maximize your fitness return? Going through mindless motions is not as effective as a sincere and concentrated effort. Developing this attitude will make the time you spend exercising more productive and enjoyable.

11. Avoid missing workouts. Feel at least a tinge of guilt when you let your commitment to workouts slide, but feel comfortable about missing a few workouts when injury or sickness require it.

12. Feel good after a workout. If you don't feel a positive postexercise glow, you are unlikely to continue. Being a little tired from a "champion" effort will help you feel good!

Motivation is only effective when the goal is meaningful and fits the individual. Once you've set your personal goals, remember to break a long-term goal—such as losing 20 pounds or running a marathon 10 minutes faster than your previous best—into more manageable goals. These not only are more likely to be realistic, but will also allow you to achieve one goal (short-term) while keeping the next within reach.

KEY POINT

Always remember to emphasize the goal of progress, not perfection!

Sample Fitness Goal Tracking Form (short-term)

Goal type (circle one):   (Short-term)   Mid-term   Long-term

Goal: Stop missing workouts for frivolous reasons. Commit!

Date goal set: 6/15

Date you'd like to accomplish goal: 6/25

Date goal accomplished: Action steps in place 6/20. Yes!! I'm on my way!

Plan of attack for accomplishing my goal:

1. Call Mary and commit to exercising with her on Monday, Wednesday, and Friday at 6:30 A.M. Schedule two appointments per week with my personal trainer on Tuesday and Thursday at 8:00 A.M.

2. Plan recreational activities with my kids and spouse on the weekends and two nights per week. Emphasize fun and active time with my family.

3. Cut out mindless channel surfing on the TV.

Goal reevaluation and change from first writing:

It might be more realistic to expect that it would take at least six months to establish a committed relationship with a training partner and integrate personal training sessions and family recreational activity into your daily schedule.

Sample Fitness Goal Tracking Form (mid-term)

Goal type (circle one):   Short-term   (Mid-term)   Long-term

Goal: Finish in top third of San Diego short-course triathlon field

Date goal set: 2/20

Date you'd like to accomplish goal: 8/16

Date goal accomplished: 8/16

Plan of attack for accomplishing my goal:

As soon as weather permits, move my indoor cycle and run training outside. Enter six short-course triathlons to give me race experience and to use as race pace/sharpening training sessions. Periodize my program to emphasize running, cycling, and swimming, but maintain my strength and flexibility with traditional stretch and strength programs. Join an organized swim program to strengthen my weakest event and get some coaching lessons from the local professional triathlete coach. Use heart rate to monitor potential overuse symptoms as I increase the duration and intensity of my workouts. Keep it FUN!

Goal reevaluation and change from first writing:

If your goal isn't attainable or realistic, create a new goal. Don't set yourself up for failure because you weren't willing to adjust the initial goal-writing effort or because of unrealistic good intentions.

If the goal had been to complete an Ironman triathlon six months from the starting date, a realistic adjustment to the goal would be to compete in short-course triathlons for the current season and lay the foundation of training necessary to complete an Ironman triathlon in the fall of the following year.

Fitness Goal Tracking Form

Goal type (circle one):   Short-term   Mid-term   Long-term

Goal: _____

Date goal set: _____

Date you'd like to accomplish goal: _____

Date goal accomplished: _____

Plan of attack for accomplishing my goal:

_____

_____

_____

_____

Goal reevaluation and change from first writing:

_____

_____

BALANCE YOUR WORKOUTS

Your Personal Trainer is a complete guide to designing your personal fitness program. It is comprehensive with regard to helping you design a fitness program that meets all of your needs and with creating a balanced approached to your program design. To get a real training advantage and the best results, it's important that you implement all the areas of fitness talked about in the following chapters.

Now that you've set the stage by defining and understanding the goals you want and need to accomplish, it's time to focus on the big three (we're not talking automakers here): cardiovascular conditioning, muscular strength and endurance, and flexibility training. Not to be forgotten are good eating habits and proper nutrition. All of these key components of fitness must be addressed correctly to ensure a balanced approach to your health and fitness.

Within each component, you likewise balance fitness. For example, in the cardiovascular component it's a good idea to use a variety of aerobic exercise choices to make your heart stronger and decrease your risk for heart disease. In strength training, it's important to work opposing muscle groups so that you create muscular balance and a pleasing physical look to your body.

KEY POINT

Balanced physical programming walks a fine line between listening to what you want to do and incorporating those interests into a program that also contains what you need to do from a total wellness perspective.

SCHEDULE YOUR WORKOUTS

Scheduling is critical to the success of your workout program. Put simply, scheduling means commitment, and commitment means success. Write your workouts in your appointment book and honor it as an important covenant. This commitment should be viewed no differently than a meeting with your boss or a prospective customer. It should not be easily erased, rescheduled, or, heaven forbid, canceled.

Over the many years that I have trained clients, the number one reason the majority of my clients train with me year after year, according to them, is that our relationship requires them to schedule and commit to an appointment. Sure, they like the fact that I motivate them, change their programs, give them new information, encourage and listen to them, but let me risk being repetitive by saying it again: the number one reason their programs are successful is that they engrave this commitment into their appointment books with indelible ink and rarely miss the opportunity to work out, feel better, and continue to receive great results!

You've got all the important information you need in this book to create the best possible program, so go ahead and write in your workout times. Go ahead, just do it!

When is the best time to work out? Don't let this question throw you. Forget about metabolism, circadian and biological rhythms, and your body's daily ups and downs. Simply etch the time in stone when it best coexists with your personality (if you hate rising early, forget about scheduling early morning workouts) and other personal commitments. Use the Weekly Workout Schedule Planning Sheet on page 36 to schedule your workouts. Be sure to transfer them to your daily planning book or carry the planning sheet with you.

> **KEY POINT**
>
> The best time to work out is the time at which you'll get it done!

PERIODIZATION MADE EASY

It's hard to embrace a word that's hard to pronounce and that many individuals do not fully comprehend. But, periodization is an important planning process that will give your training new life, and it's easy to do.

A periodized program varies how hard, how much, and how often you train and the types of activity you train with over specific time periods. Periodization encourages you to introduce purposeful change and variety into your program plans.

> **KEY POINT**
>
> Periodization is probably most simply defined as "planned results."

Most fitness articles mention, and most fitness professionals claim, that periodization should be incorporated into every program-planning process.

Sample Weekly Workout Schedule Planning Sheet

Week of: __6/10-6/16__

Monday	Tuesday	Wednesday	Thursday	Friday	Saturday	Sunday
With whom: Mary	With whom: John, my personal trainer	With whom: Mary	With whom: John, my personal trainer	With whom: Mary	With whom: Family	With whom: Family
Where: Meet at park	Where: Gym	Where: Meet at park	Where: Gym	Where: Meet at park	Where: Hike and soccer	Where: Rest day
A.M.	**A.M.**	**A.M.**	**A.M.**	**A.M.**	**A.M.**	**A.M.**
5:00	5:00	5:00	5:00	5:00	5:00	5:00
(6:00)	6:00	(6:00)	6:00	(6:00)	6:00	6:00
7:00	7:00	7:00	7:00	7:00	7:00	7:00
8:00	8:00	8:00	8:00/	8:00	8:00	8:00
9:00	9:00	9:00	9:00	9:00	9:00	9:00
10:00	10:00	10:00	10:00	10:00	(10:00)	10:00
11:00	11:00	11:00	11:00	11:00	11:00	11:00
P.M.	**P.M.**	**P.M.**	**P.M.**	**P.M.**	**P.M.**	**P.M.**
12:00	12:00	12:00	12:00	12:00	12:00	12:00
1:00	1:00	1:00	1:00	1:00	1:00	1:00
2:00	2:00	2:00	2:00	2:00	2:00	2:00
3:00	3:00	3:00	3:00	3:00	3:00	3:00
4:00	4:00	4:00	4:00	4:00	(4:00)	4:00
5:00	5:00	5:00	5:00	5:00	5:00	5:00
6:00	(6:00)	6:00	(6:00)	6:00	6:00	6:00
7:00	7:00	7:00	7:00	7:00	7:00	7:00
8:00	8:00	8:00	8:00	8:00	8:00	8:00
9:00	9:00	9:00	9:00	9:00	9:00	9:00

Weekly Workout Schedule Planning Sheet

Week of: _____

Monday	Tuesday	Wednesday	Thursday	Friday	Saturday	Sunday
With whom:	With whom:	With whom:	With whom:	With whom:	With whom:	With whom:
Where:	Where:	Where:	Where:	Where:	Where:	Where:
A.M.	**A.M.**	**A.M.**	**A.M.**	**A.M.**	**A.M.**	**A.M.**
5:00	5:00	5:00	5:00	5:00	5:00	5:00
6:00	6:00	6:00	6:00	6:00	6:00	6:00
7:00	7:00	7:00	7:00	7:00	7:00	7:00
8:00	8:00	8:00	8:00	8:00	8:00	8:00
9:00	9:00	9:00	9:00	9:00	9:00	9:00
10:00	10:00	10:00	10:00	10:00	10:00	10:00
11:00	11:00	11:00	11:00	11:00	11:00	11:00
P.M.	**P.M.**	**P.M.**	**P.M.**	**P.M.**	**P.M.**	**P.M.**
12:00	12:00	12:00	12:00	12:00	12:00	12:00
1:00	1:00	1:00	1:00	1:00	1:00	1:00
2:00	2:00	2:00	2:00	2:00	2:00	2:00
3:00	3:00	3:00	3:00	3:00	3:00	3:00
4:00	4:00	4:00	4:00	4:00	4:00	4:00
5:00	5:00	5:00	5:00	5:00	5:00	5:00
6:00	6:00	6:00	6:00	6:00	6:00	6:00
7:00	7:00	7:00	7:00	7:00	7:00	7:00
8:00	8:00	8:00	8:00	8:00	8:00	8:00
9:00	9:00	9:00	9:00	9:00	9:00	9:00

While there is quite a bit of information in reference to periodization training developed for elite athletes, these programs are very technical, highly specific, focus on "peaking" for athletic performance, and are often confusing since no one standard approach exists. Few, if any, formulas exist that explain how to incorporate a periodized program into simple fitness routines without investing hours of planning. However, *Your Personal Trainer* provides you with an easy-to-use model.

By manipulating volume of work (i.e., reps, sets, duration) and intensity of effort, and by strategically placing rest, maintenance, and recovery phases in the overall periodization plan, you can easily transfer complex concepts of periodization to fitness goals. These include weight management, increased muscle strength, improvement in cardiovascular fitness, and improvement in your times in a 10K running race.

Periodization has the potential to

- promote optimal response to the training stimulus or work effort,
- decrease the potential for overuse injuries,
- keep you fresh and progressing toward your ultimate training goal(s),
- optimize your personal efforts, and
- enhance compliance.

Principles of Periodization

Periodization is a method to organize training. It cycles volume (reps, sets, minutes, distance, duration) and intensity (load, force, weight lifted, speed) over specific time periods. Periodization may be viewed from two perspectives. One perspective is to use an activity or sport by itself to develop fitness, enhance health, or improve performance. A second approach uses the activity or sport, along with other nonspecific cross-training activities, to develop fitness and improve performance while simultaneously keeping the training progressing.

Considerable scientific research and experience shows that the second system—using sport movement and supplementary training that includes a variety of cardiovascular, muscular strength and endurance, and flexibility conditioning—is far more effective than training with one fixed set of activity skills or sport alone. The underlying science is related to optimal stress or intensity, and restoration or recovery. In other words, work (exercise) must be followed by rest. Of these key aspects—intensity and recovery—one is not better than the other. Each must be given equal emphasis and preferential time.

Comparing Athletes to Fitness Enthusiasts

The most obvious difference between elite athletes and most fitness participants is that the need to "peak" for performance is minimal or nonexistent for the latter. For the athlete, maximal performance generally coincides with important competitions. Thus, the change from one phase of training to another will be more subtle for fitness training than for the high-level athlete. For the average client, training phases translate to (1) preparation or buildup, (2) goal attainment, and (3) restoration/recovery. For most active people who have achieved a desirable level of fitness, the goal may be variety of activity, solidifying current fitness levels, and establishing commitment to exercise on a regular basis.

KEY POINT

Ongoing evaluation of your needs and goals is a necessity, whether you're just starting an exercise program or have attained a high level of fitness.

A well-planned periodized program looks at short-term, mid-term, and long-term needs. Such a planning process considers daily workouts (microcycles of about 7 to 10 days), an agenda that accounts for three to four weeks of training (mesocycles), and an overall annual scheme, or at least several months of planning (macrocycle). After every three to four weeks of progressive overload, insert at least several workouts of active recovery. Active recovery, or active rest, is usually performed at lower intensities of effort and duration than previous exercise levels. Also, you should consider using different activities (cross-training) at least part of the time during this recovery and restoration time period.

When planned results are achieved, the intensity of effort or load is determined for the next phase. Generally, unless entering into a restoration phase or ending a mesocycle of three to four weeks, the sequence of the preceding workouts is repeated at higher intensity levels. This cyclic process will determine the contents and organization of the programming process.

Figure 2.1 illustrates a progressive overload pattern using active rest after each three- to four-week mesocycle. The beginning of each new mesocycle should be started at a lower intensity than that used in the last week of the previous mesocycle.

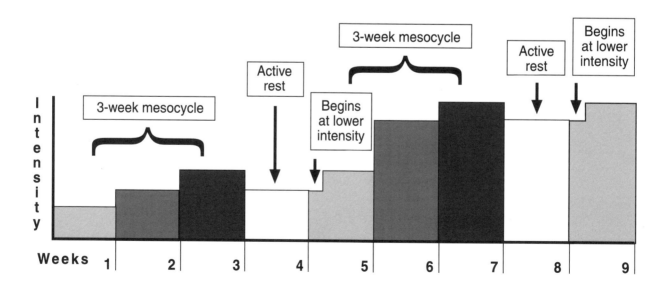

Figure 2.1 Applying periodization will help your workouts.

Periodization Model for Health and Fitness

To the fitness professional, periodization means varying workouts over set time periods to optimize performance and fitness gains. Follow these steps to plan a progressive, goal-oriented training program that achieves superb results.

Step 1: Set the Goal(s)
- Cardiovascular goals
- Muscular strength and endurance goals
- Flexibility goals
- Other goals (e.g., set a new PR—your personal record or best—in your next 10K race or prepare for a two-week backpacking trip)

Step 2: Determine How to Achieve the Goal(s)
- Assess time availability
- Identify types (modes) of activity
- Match training to goals
- Choose activities that you like

Step 3: Identify Training Phases and Create an Exercise Plan
- Training phases

   Develop 3- to 10-day short-term planning (microcycle).

   Develop a three- to four-week training plan (mesocycle).

   Develop a yearly organizational training plan (macrocycle), or at least three to four months of mesocycles.

   Plan a general preparation phase of three to four weeks (one mesocycle), which may repeat several times.
- Exercise plan

   Manipulate frequency, intensity, and duration of each activity for specific results in the body's energy and physiologic systems.

   Apply appropriate frequency, intensity, and duration principles to each fitness component in the general preparation and goal phase.

   Control results by proper intensity of effort (load) and adequate recovery (restoration).

Step 4: Plan Volume and Intensity (Overload)
- Vary volume and overload on a cyclic basis

   Change volume and overload every three to four weeks at least, and possibly within a 3- to 10-day microcycle.

   Plan to increase or decrease volume and intensity.

   Use lower intensities and less duration during restoration (active rest).

   Start the new mesocycle after active recovery at a slightly lower intensity than the previous cycle.

- Allow for the restoration/recovery process

  Generally, do not increase progressive overload for more than three to four continuous weeks.

  Follow any sustained, progressive three- to four-week (mesocycle) increase in overload with at least several days of active recovery at a lower intensity. The effort is less intense when compared to the last overload phase in which you participated (see figure 2.1 on page 38).

  After active recovery, start the new mesocycle at a slightly lower intensity than the previous cycle (see figure 2.1).

  Remember, the key to optimal results is not a steady, relentless increase in intensity over long periods of time.

Step 5: Regularly Evaluate the Periodization Planning Process
- Monitor results and progress
- Use fitness assessment (optional)
- Recognize goal achievement
- Observe your compliance and enthusiasm toward the program

Case Study: From Theory to Your Program

Let's apply these principles to the program of a hypothetical exerciser. Jenna is a new exerciser and her goals are weight loss, weight management, and "increased energy level." Jenna understands that a long-term plan (macrocycle) will focus on important fitness components that will help her realize her training goals.

1.   Set the Goals

A good first step in creating a periodized program is to assess Jenna's current fitness levels in categories related to her goals of weight loss, weight management, and increased energy. Fitness testing will establish a reference point for comparing fitness improvements over time. This is one way to evaluate the effectiveness of a planning program.

2.   Determine How to Achieve the Goals

Improvements in cardiovascular fitness and muscular strength and endurance will be very important to help Jenna attain her goals. She understands the important contribution cardiovascular fitness gives to calorie burning and knows that if she becomes more fit, she will be able to burn more calories and fat. She also will develop greater endurance, which could lead to a feeling of "more energy."

Strength training will enhance Jenna's feelings of personal power and control. Because gains in muscle strength increase muscle endurance, she will have new energy and strength at the end of the day. Also, increases in lean muscle mass will "reshape" her body and increase her resting metabolic rate, which will help her lose body fat and maintain her new, desirable weight.

> ### KEY POINT
>
> Part of the key to attaining goals is to create an environment in which you have a sense of ownership (a feeling that "this is what I want to do") and personal responsibility, and an understanding of why a specific approach is being organized and planned. This feeling of ownership and responsibility can be realized only through education and feeling as though you're on the right track.

After talking about her goals, it became clear that Jenna wanted to accomplish her goals with a multi-activity approach.

3.   Identify Training Phases and Create an Exercise Plan

It is usually unrealistic to plan an entire year and expect to stick to it. Instead, stay focused on microcycles and mesocycles. This will save valuable time when one of life's events inevitably necessitates a major change in your training program or schedule.

   a. Over a 3- to 10-day microcycle, plan a menu of workouts that fit into the session.

   b. Extend the microcycle to a planned three- to four-week mesocycle.

   c. A "mini" macrocycle of three to four months (long-term planning) is the next step.

Since Jenna is new to fitness and her goals are set, her first two months (two mesocycles) of training will consist of about six to seven 3- to 10-day microcycles. These microcycles will focus on a preparation phase that reflects the goals of increased overall endurance ("energy") and weight management. Her program initially shapes up like this:

   a. A series of six or seven microcycles (about two months) emphasizing a basic, but progressive, resistance and cardiovascular program. This series of microcycles is equivalent to two mesocycles. (Each mesocycle is about three to four weeks in length.)

   b. After the first mesocycle (three to four weeks), active rest should be used for about three to five workouts.

   c. A second mesocycle will emphasize continued, progressive increases in intensity. If Jenna is ready, exercise variety will be introduced within each fitness component.

4.   Plan Volume and Intensity

After the preparation phase is well established (in about eight weeks), the third mesocycle begins and progresses to the goal phase. This cycle emphasizes a hypertrophy phase (increased muscle size) for strength and continued challenges in duration and intensity of effort for cardiovascular conditioning. For example, Jenna may have progressed from a 12- to 20-repetition overload to fatigue to an 8- to 12-repetition overload to fatigue. Since the first two mesocycles built the base of aerobic endurance, the third mesocycle will incorporate intervals, and intensity, duration, and frequency will be manipulated.

The goal of these specific time periods is to provide an overload that is challenging, progressive, and appropriate to Jenna's new fitness gains.

Micro- and mesocycles also create goals that are reasonable, and most important, attainable in short time frames. This keeps Jenna motivated, helps her stick to her exercise program, and keeps her physiologically fresh.

After the completion of this third mesocycle, active rest will be used, including a variety of cross-training activities. Jenna will experience different cardio conditioning activities, will change strength exercises, or will switch to entirely different (unrelated) activity during this active recovery.

> ## KEY POINT
>
> Remember, active recovery is performed at lower intensities of effort (and usually with less quantity or duration) than in previous micro- or mesocycle time periods. Active recovery allows for physical recovery and enhancement of the adaptation process. Effort is 50 percent of the training equation, and recovery/restoration is the other important half!

5. Evaluate the Program

Reassessment of Jenna's goals, results, interest, and enthusiasm can never happen too often. This keeps an open and fresh connection with Jenna's needs and wants and continues to help her ask the question, "Where should I go from here?"

Implementing Periodized Fitness

The key to successful periodization is your ability to create challenges to the body with new activities and progressive overload (intensity).

Applying Periodization to Fitness Results

1. Determine and select goal(s).
2. Determine and assess starting fitness level (optional, see chapter 1).
3. Develop a 3- to 10-day menu (microcycle) of daily workouts.
4. Develop a 3- to 4-week menu (mesocycle) of daily workouts.
5. Develop a 4-month menu (modified macrocycle) of workouts.
6. Develop at least four mesocycles (12-16 weeks of workouts). Four mesocycles could be considered as a "mini" macrocycle.
7. Reevaluate goals, progress, and effectiveness of the program after each daily workout, and especially after each 3- or 4-week mesocycle.
8. Plan and organize a recovery or restoration phase, consisting of at least several workouts, after every mesocycle (3-4 weeks). Utilize the concept of active rest. Active rest encourages the participant to engage in different activities, preferably at lower intensities. This "unloading" phase is critical to optimizing results and minimizing injury potential.
9. Make sure you exercise at the right intensity or level of effort for each fitness component. Intensity should reflect your personal fitness level and personal goals.
10. Develop an individual exercise plan. When developing meso- or macrocycles, make sure that all necessary fitness components are included in the planning process and emphasized in the right amounts (frequency, duration) and intensity to move you toward the accomplishment of your goals.

Sample Weekly Workout Planning Sheet Week Of: 6/10-6/16

Aerobic Exercise	Strength Exercise	Stretching Exercise
Type of aerobic exercises:	**Body part targeted**	**Body part targeted**
Monday: easy jog Tuesday: indoor cycling Wednesday: hard run Thursday: swim Friday: moderate run Saturday: strolling with family in park Sunday: REST	☑ chest ☑ back ☑ lats ☑ arms ☑ shoulders ☑ abs ☑ back ☑ upper legs ☑ lower legs ☑ rotator cuff ❑ other _____ ❑ other _____ ❑ other _____ ❑ other _____ ❑ other _____	☑ chest ☑ back ☑ lats ☑ arms ☑ shoulders ☑ abs ☑ back ☑ upper legs ☑ lower legs ☑ rotator cuff ❑ other _____ ❑ other _____ ❑ other _____ ❑ other _____ ❑ other _____
How often? **(3-6 times per week)**	**How often?** **(at least 2 times per week)**	**How often?** **(at least each time you workout)**
Monday: ☑ Tuesday: ☑ Wednesday: ☑ Thursday: ☑ Friday: ☑ Saturday: ☑ Sunday: ❑	Monday: ❑ Tuesday: ☑ Wednesday: ❑ Thursday: ☑ Friday: ❑ Saturday: ❑ Sunday: ❑	Monday: ☑ Tuesday: ☑ Wednesday: ☑ Thursday: ☑ Friday: ☑ Saturday: ☑ Sunday: ❑
How hard? **(use RPE* and heart rate)**	**Reps / sets / loads**	**How hard?**
Monday: RPE of 3-4 HR* 50-60% of HRR* Tuesday: RPE 4-5	(see table below)	To the point of tension or "comfortably uncomfortable"

Strength Exercise — Reps / sets / loads:

	Reps	Sets	Load
Monday:			
Tuesday:	12-15	2	70% of 1 RM*

continued

Sample Weekly Workout Planning Sheet *(continued)*

How hard? (use RPE* and heart rate)		Reps / sets / loads				How hard?
			Reps	Sets	Load	
Wed:	RPE of 4-8 Peak HR of 80-85% of HRR	Wed:				To the point of tension or "comfortably uncomfortable"
Thurs:	RPE 4-5	Thurs:	6-8	3	80-85% of 1 RM	
Fri:	RPE of 4-5 No HR monitoring	Fri:				
Sat:	Unstructural	Sat:				
Sun:		Sun:				

How long?		How long?	Length of hold?
Mon:	50 minutes depending on the number of exercises, reps, sets, and loads	Generally, 20-60 minutes, hold, no bouncing	10 to 60 seconds with static
Tues:	20 minutes		
Wed:	30 minutes of interval 15 minutes of warm-up and cool-down		Number of repetitions and holds per stretch: generally, 1-3 per body part
Thurs:	20 minutes		
Fri:	35 minutes		
Sat:	unstructured		
Sun:			

*HR = heart rate; RPE = rate of perceived exertion; HRR = heart rate reserve; RM = repetition max

---

KEY POINT

If your body is constantly challenged, it will keep responding, your mind will stay inspired, and your risk of overuse injury will decrease.

Just as your body experiences the peak benefits of one mesocycle of planned workouts and starts to adapt to it, you move into a whole new three- to four-week cycle that offers an entirely new set of challenges.

Management and organization of your program involves your awareness of what drives and motivates you. Within a 24-hour period, your perceptions of fatigue, strength, and motivation may vary, so it is helpful to be aware of influences that will challenge you to adapt your planning.

Weekly Workout Planning Sheet Week Of: _____

Aerobic Exercise	Strength Exercise	Stretching Exercise
Type of aerobic exercises:	**Body part targeted**	**Body part targeted**
Monday: Tuesday: Wednesday: Thursday: Friday: Saturday: Sunday:	❏ chest ❏ back ❏ lats ❏ arms ❏ shoulders ❏ abs ❏ back ❏ upper legs ❏ lower legs ❏ rotator cuff ❏ other _____ ❏ other _____ ❏ other _____ ❏ other _____ ❏ other _____	❏ chest ❏ back ❏ lats ❏ arms ❏ shoulders ❏ abs ❏ back ❏ upper legs ❏ lower legs ❏ rotator cuff ❏ other _____ ❏ other _____ ❏ other _____ ❏ other _____ ❏ other _____
How often? **(3-6 times per week)**	**How often?** **(at least 2 times per week)**	**How often?** **(at least each time you workout)**
Monday: ❏ Tuesday: ❏ Wednesday: ❏ Thursday: ❏ Friday: ❏ Saturday: ❏ Sunday: ❏	Monday: ❏ Tuesday: ❏ Wednesday: ❏ Thursday: ❏ Friday: ❏ Saturday: ❏ Sunday: ❏	Monday: ❏ Tuesday: ❏ Wednesday: ❏ Thursday: ❏ Friday: ❏ Saturday: ❏ Sunday: ❏
How hard? **(use RPE* and heart rate)**	**Reps / sets / loads**	**How hard?**
Monday: Tuesday:	Monday: <u>Reps</u> <u>Sets</u> <u>Load</u> Tuesday:	To the point of tension or "comfortably uncomfortable"

continued

Weekly Workout Planning Sheet *(continued)*

How hard? (use RPE* and heart rate)	Rep / sets / loads	How hard?
Wednesday: Thursday: Friday: Saturday: Sunday:	Wednesday: Thursday: Friday: Saturday: Sunday:	
How long?	**How long?**	**Length of hold?**
Monday: Tuesday: Wednesday: Thursday: Friday: Saturday: Sunday:	Generally, 20-60 minutes, depending on the number of exercises, reps, sets, and loads	10 to 60 seconds with static hold, no bouncing Number of repetitions and holds per stretch: generally, 1-3

*HR = heart rate; RPE = rate of perceived exertion; HRR = heart rate reserve; RM = repetition max

Tracking Your Periodized Program

You can track a periodized program in several ways. One idea is to label a manila folder with each mesocycle and keep your Weekly Workout Planning Sheets in the folders. Then place 4 to 12 manila file folders (representing 4 to 12 mesocycles) inside a hanging file folder. You can organize the same system on your computer by creating a file for each mesocycle and placing programs in it (consider scanning or inputting the data from the Weekly Workout Planning Sheet into your computer). The Periodization Planning Worksheet is a model that you may want to follow as you develop your own record-keeping system (page 47). It gives you a more general, quick look at your weekly periodized program over a time frame that represents two mesocycles.

It is obvious that periodization, planning, and program organization are not inherently complex. However, planning does require some forethought and a reasonable time investment. On the other hand, it is well worth that investment, since periodization makes you accountable for results. Because the process involves management, planning, and organization, it is results oriented. And you win!

REALITY CHECK

Well-known sports medicine expert Dr. Randy Eichner calls self-delusion the "most popular indoor sport" (*Sports Medicine Digest*, December 1993). What

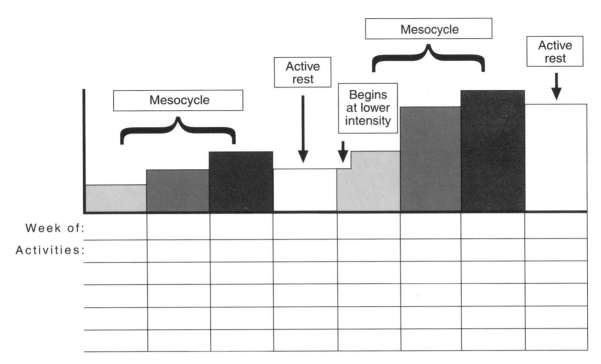

Figure 2.2   Periodization planning worksheet.

he's getting at is that most of us overestimate how much we exercise and underestimate how much we eat. While weight maintenance and weight loss are very complex, for example, part of the reason that some obese people can't lose weight, according to Dr. Eichner, is self-delusion. He refers to a sophisticated study that reports that in a failed diet group, subjects ate 1,000 calories more than they recorded in their diaries and burned 250 fewer calories than their exercise records indicated.

Interestingly, this same pattern is seen in young, old, fat, or slim people (that's where all of us fit in!). Four out of five people believe that they eat less and exercise more than they actually do (Eichner, 1993). Remember, regardless of your goal, regardless of what you write down, results depend on what you do, not on what you believe you are doing.

Quick Index:

3 Target the Right Equipment

Rarely are workout space and equipment the determining factors with regard to great training results. Probably the most important factor is how much effort you put into your workout, or how often and how long you work out. In later chapters, *Your Personal Trainer* will show you how to train smart! But, while place and equipment availability don't make or break a program, they can have a big impact if you choose poorly. It is encouraging to know that many simple solutions exist when you are confronted with limited equipment options. On the other hand, working in a well-equipped gym and pleasing environment does not guarantee a successful training outcome. Your decision about how you work out, where you work out, and what equipment you use should be made only after doing your homework. *Your Personal Trainer* supplies the answers.

WORKING OUT AT THE GYM

Working out in a public gym environment has received both rave reviews and harsh criticism. Here are the questions to ask yourself: Is the gym right for you? Does the social environment motivate or distract you? Is the excitement and noise a call to action or a bombardment to your senses? Does being around other exercisers (many of whom are buffed or scantily clad) encourage or intimidate you?

A health club or fitness studio can provide a place to work out and most likely offers a diversity of equipment options that can help you create a balanced, varied, and interesting program. Instruction from qualified fitness professionals may also be available. Gym workouts can also complement activities you do outside the club.

If your impression of the public gym is that of a crowded and far-away fitness factory, you might be one of the increasing number of people who are opting to bypass the crowds and stay fit by setting up a gym at home. If you're thinking that the initiation fee and monthly dues are resulting in nothing more substantial than a chance to visit a gym that is too loud, and burdened with too many sweating, competitive people who are waiting in line to push and pull against resistance or run nowhere on a treadmill, you're ready for a home gym.

Why not invest your money in a permanent return? A personal gym might serve you better by allowing you to work out in the convenient, private, and time-saving atmosphere of home sweet home!

WORKING OUT AT HOME

If the goosebumps and anxiety are just starting to fade after reading the previous section, you're probably thinking that working out in the privacy of your home is indeed a great idea, for no better reasons than saving time and personal sanity. Plus, there's no crowded prime time in my home gym. (Beware: unless your hectic home life invades!)

Just because you exercise at home doesn't mean you can't still belong to a health club. A recent study by the Fitness Products Council showed that 63 percent of exercisers who belonged to a health club also exercised with equipment in their homes. In the same study, 43 percent of Americans surveyed said they didn't exercise regularly because of time constraints (reported in *ACE FitnessMatters*, Vol. 3, No. 1: January/February, 1997).

KEY POINT

The opportunity to work out needs to be available at every turn in your daily schedule. It makes sense to be committed to exercise in a variety of ways that makes exercise easy, accessible, and convenient. At every turn, the chance to agitate your body on a regular basis should be underfoot!

Creating a Home Gym

Creating a home gym, if approached correctly, is easy and satisfying. Joining a health club requires you to check out the facility, equipment options, and staff, but it's pretty easy to come to an informed decision as to whether the club is right for you. Likewise, you need to do some earnest homework and consider some important questions before you establish your "Fitness Palace."

Locate the Right Exercise Space

Wherever you decide to place your home gym, it should be a comfortable and inviting area. You can create a superb gym regardless of whether it is located in a small studio apartment, townhouse, condominium, home office, or an estate. But, if it's cramped, dim, drab, dingy, or stuffy, this isn't a place you're going to want to spend time. If it's bright, organized, uncluttered, fresh, and attractive, it's a lot easier to get excited about exercising.

Natural light from windows and skylights works best to motivate exercise spirit, and windows and skylights can provide a visual distraction. Walls and mirrors can take you only so far. (Some days, you just don't want to look at yourself or that picture of some "hard body" on the wall.) If the space you've chosen is dark, or you work out at night, provide enough artificial lighting so that you aren't lulled into thinking you're at a romantic, candlelit dinner or mired in a dungeon. Make sure you have an option for fresh air ventilation, if possible. As a minimum, air circulation should be provided by a heating and cooling system or portable fans. You'll appreciate the right lighting and refreshing air in all seasons. Remember, you're there to breathe deeply and work out, and you need a gym environment that proves irresistible!

Hardwood floors are an ideal surface on which to place equipment. They are stable and easy to clean. Their downside is that they scratch easily and are noisier. (This is especially important to consider if you have family members or neighbors who don't appreciate your early or late night exercise enthusiasm!) To protect wood floors and ease the noise concern, rubber mats (some interlock into a myriad of configurations) are available and specially designed to fit beneath exercise equipment or cover an entire area. If you use carpeting or a rug, a short-pile indoor-outdoor cut is the best. It should be of commercial (heavy-duty) quality and have little or no padding underneath. Equipment can leave an almost permanent imprint on thickly padded surfaces, which can create a less stable exercising surface. If you exercise on the floor, use an exercise mat to protect the carpeting from sweat and cushion your body. Choose carpet color combinations that will not show dirt, machinery oil, or foot traffic patterns.

Mirrors not only help you check your exercise form and posture, but if placed correctly, can turn a small area into a seemingly larger space. Mirrors can help create a feeling of openness and a sense of spaciousness when it does not physically exist. A four- by six- to eight-foot mirror placed horizontally on a wall and about 18 inches from the floor can totally recreate the atmosphere of any exercise area.

Finally, it's nice to consider the positive aspect (or is it distraction?) of watching TV and listening to music while exercising. You can use your cordless phone, too. The obvious attraction for many is distraction and the fact that you can accomplish at least two or three tasks simultaneously in a time slot designated for your exercise. For example, you can get your exercise in, call a couple of friends, and keep an ear tuned to your favorite TV show. To the purist this may seem like a cop-out, but if time is at a premium, it helps you pass the time, you're seeing the results you want, and it keeps exercising FUN—do it!

HOME EQUIPMENT PURCHASES

Here's a primer on how to go about selecting your home gym equipment. Before you look at the Home Gym Pre-Assessment Questionnaire and the Checklist for Home Equipment Purchases, plant the following thought firmly in your brain: regardless of how big or small your home gym is, whether you have an entire room or a corner spot dedicated, try to minimize the necessity of taking down and setting up equipment.

Let me state it more strongly. Forget it! It doesn't work! More programs and good intentions fall short because of a failure to commit space to allow for permanent setup of equipment. Having to set up and take down equipment gives you another excuse for not exercising. If space is at a premium in your home, realize that you don't need a lot of this precious commodity to set up a gym. If you shop smart, you can buy equipment that fits into small spaces nicely, is versatile enough to offer more than one type of exercise, and won't compromise the effectiveness and safety of your workout.

Home Gym Pre-Assessment Questionnaire

• What fitness activities have I found to be successful?_____

• What fitness activities do I find fun and enjoyable and will likely continue for my lifetime?_____

_____

• What types of fitness equipment have I used and enjoyed in the past?_____

_____

• What, if any, physical limitations do I have (problems such as a bad back, knees, shoulders, wrists, or arthritis)?_____

How would equipment choices complement, or possibly exacerbate, this condition? _____

_____

• Are my short- and long-term goals in line with what I am considering purchasing?   Yes   No

If yes, how will the equipment purchased help me accomplish my goals?

_____

• Will my equipment selections allow me to create balanced workout options that target the major components of fitness, including cardiovascular conditioning, muscular strength and endurance, and flexibility training? If so, how?_____

_____

• Does my home gym equipment offer me the option of cross-training and variety? If so, how?

_____

• Will anyone else in my household be using the equipment? If so, will my equipment selection meet their goals and allow them to exercise safely? Will children be using the equipment?

_____

• Am I willing to dedicate space in my home for my home gym? If so, have I thought about electrical prerequisites (most home-version cardio machines use standard wall outlets), weight requirements, lighting needs, and floor surfaces?_____

_____

> **KEY POINT**
>
> Everyone hypes the idea of storing equipment, but it doesn't get used when it's under your bed or in a closet!

Aerobic Equipment

The simplest and least expensive cardiovascular equipment is a good pair of walking, running, or cross-training shoes. Regardless of how you strengthen your heart, you'll probably need at least a couple of pairs of good "treads" to complement the cardio activity you participate in. Different activities often require different shoes, and your shoes need time to air out before the next workout. So, it's a good idea to visit a high-end specialty shoe store if you don't know the types of shoes you need for your workouts.

Some examples of the more popular cardiovascular equipment you have to choose from are treadmills, steppers/climbers, elliptical trainers, ski machines, lateral trainers (side-to-side pushing or sliding movement), manual resistance stationary cycles, electronic stationary cycles (i.e., programmable and usually an upright sitting position), recumbent bikes, and rowing machines. Note that the stationary cycle or spin-training craze warrants that you try the new breed of high-performance "spin" training bikes. This newer breed of spin-training bikes is more fully adjustable to your body's dimensions, but try before you buy! Stationary bikes have come a long way.

Many safety features, different types of electronics, and optional upgrade choices are available on this huge selection of choices. Your choice really comes down to a personal decision (what do you love to do?) and variety.

> **KEY POINT**
>
> Contrary to what you hear, no one cardiovascular machine or activity is better than the other when calorie expenditure, fat burning, and physical conditioning benefits are compared. How long, how hard, and how often you exercise can easily be adjusted on all of the pieces of cardio equipment listed, to be comparable with any other cardiovascular conditioning activity.

Remember the truism "know thyself". Find several activities you really enjoy and purchase a couple of pieces of equipment so you can cross-train indoors when necessary. Probably the most solid choice you can make is to purchase a fully automated treadmill. (If you despise walking or running on treadmills, forget this recommendation!) Complement this choice with a manual resistance bike, climber/stepper, or rowing machine. Cross-training between aerobic exercises will keep you from getting bored out of your head and provide new physiological stimulation. You can even create a sport conditioning circuit. This type of approach will keep you enthusiastic about exercise and keep you from hitting exercise plateaus and falling into an exercise rut. Remember, you can exercise outdoors, too!

Checklist for Home Equipment Purchases

This checklist will encourage you to think about information you should consider before buying home fitness equipment. Put a check mark next to each question to which your answer is yes. If you check off the majority of questions in the list, you're on your way to making an informed and useful choice.

❏ Will I look to a "specialty fitness retailer" or qualified fitness professional to assist me in the research and selection of my home fitness equipment? (Specialty fitness retailers usually have more qualified sales personnel than mass merchandising sporting goods chains. Additionally, many specialty retailers carry commercial grade equipment—such as the equipment clubs use that get heavy use—and high-quality home versions of this trustworthy, time-tested equipment.)

❏ Do I understand the high-tech techno talk? (If not, ask what it means, what it costs you, and how it will help your program. If you get more babble and no helpful answers, it's time to move on.)

❏ Will I consider each piece of equipment that I purchase with regard to cost, space efficiency, portability, variety, and diversity, and each of these five qualities' importance to my situation? (Purchasing a bench that declines, lies flat, and inclines is a good example of a piece of equipment that exemplifies these five qualities.)

❏ Have I tried out every piece of equipment to see if I like it? (When you shop, wear your workout shoes and comfortable clothes. Spend at least 5 to 10 minutes on every piece of equipment you're considering, and make your own adjustments after the salesperson shows you how. Many specialty retail stores will encourage you to test-ride equipment and have models set up just for this purpose. Or, you can visit local gyms and experience a variety of equipment. Many gyms offer free one-week trials you can take advantage of or you can purchase day or short-term memberships so you can try out different equipment.)

❏ Have I talked to other people who have used this equipment? (Ask the person selling the equipment to give you a list of customers who have bought that particular piece of equipment.)

❏ Will I really use this equipment or is it going to be a high-priced dust collector?

❏ Am I committed to buying quality equipment that will last me a lifetime? (This is in comparison to buying "junk" that will have to be replaced, will frustrate your exercise efforts, and may be unsafe!)

❏ Is this a piece of equipment that will stand the test time, or is it trend-influenced and destined to fall out of fashion in time? (Good examples of timeless equipment that never lose their appeal are motorized treadmills and free weights such as dumbbells.)

❏ Does an equipment purchase come with personal instruction (specialty store retailers usually have a very knowledgeable sales staff and relationships with personal trainers in your area), a videotaped workout and instruction, and other written instructional material? (Some retailers arrange a free workout with a personal trainer who can show you the ins and outs of your new equipment. Make sure the trainer is certified by a nationally recognized certifying organization.)

❏ What is the warranty for parts and labor? (Although the manufacturer's warranty is usually 90 days, ask the retailer if they'll back the equipment for a year. To get a sale, they probably will. Besides, if you're buying a quality piece of equipment, this one-year insurance is probably overkill and the store won't really be at any additional risk. So why not ask for it?)

❏ Can warranty work, part replacement, repairs, and service be performed locally, or do you have to ship the equipment? (Specialty retailers generally take care of you since they'd like your repeat business or for you to refer others to them. And, they usually have a full-service repair, delivery, and maintenance department.)

❏ Can I trade the equipment in and upgrade to a higher-quality piece?

continued

Checklist for Home Equipment Purchases *(continued)*

❏ Has the store you're considering purchasing from been in business for a number of years? (Ask the store manager if he could contact any customers who have purchased the equipment you're interested in, and who might be available to talk with you about their purchase.)

❏ Is the equipment made by a major manufacturer? (With regard to quality and equipment that will serve you for the long haul, you usually can't go wrong buying brand names.)

❏ Is the equipment quiet when in use?

❏ Is the cushioning made of dense and supportive, yet forgiving, material? Is the external upholstery covering of high quality? (Compare commercial equipment such as you see in gyms with some "cheesy" home exercise equipment and you'll see, and feel, the difference. Go for the high-grade equipment. You'll pay more and be glad you did!)

❏ Do cables and pulleys move smoothly and quietly?

❏ What are the safety features?

❏ Is the cost of delivery and installation included in the purchase price? (If not, bargain for it!)

❏ Is any assembly required after delivery? If it is necessary, is it included in the purchase price? (If it isn't, ask for it. If a lot of assembly is required, you have the potential for numerous nuts and bolts to work themselves loose over time. Look for pieces that have welded frames and joints and minimal assembly requirements.)

❏ What is the return policy? (The manufacturer or retail store should offer, at a minimum, an unconditional, 30-day return policy. If for some reason you buy equipment you haven't tried, find out the details of returning the product. Two important questions to ask are whether you have to pay return shipping and whether any of your original purchase price is nonrefundable. Can you trust the company you're buying from? A "free" 30-day trial can cost you some significant money, not to mention the hassle of repacking the junk and sending it back!)

❏ If a salesperson hurries or tries to push me into a quick decision without answering my questions and encouraging me to try the equipment, will I promptly walk out the door? (You can do this politely, and the answer should be yes.)

Strength Equipment

Don't believe it when you read, or someone tells you, that weight machines or multistation gyms are the safest. Safest compared to what? It is true you can't drop a weight on the floor, or your toe, when using these units. But, what good is this safety feature to you if you end up wrecking your shoulder because an exercise motion is incorrectly designed and you have no way to correct it, or you get into and out of a machine incorrectly and tear off your upper limbs? On the other hand, like most pieces of exercise equipment, machines aren't necessarily bad if they're used properly and designed correctly.

The previous paragraph illustrates how unfounded biases (hearsay) sometimes blind you to the big picture and can lead you astray, get you hurt, prevent you from getting the results you want, and keep you lost in the hardware jungle! Read on so you can get the whole story.

A wide variety of strength exercise equipment is available for you to train your entire body effectively. There is overlap from category to category. Strength exercise equipment includes the following:

- Free weights (Dumbbells, barbells and hand-held weights can be used to create a myriad of exercise options that are biomechanically correct.)
- Multistation weight machines (They have their pros and cons and are generally pulley/cable systems that are routed to selectorized plates or weight stacks, although some movements are limited by what the cable connects to, for example, a straight bar or chest flye attachment.)
- Pulley/cable systems (As mentioned, multistation gyms are often pulley/cable systems that use weight stacks for resistance and the cable connects to various exercise devices. Bowflex is an example of a pulley/cable system that uses composite resistance rods rather than weight stacks to produce progressive resistance, and the use of cables attached to hand grips allows you to lift correctly with unlimited exercise design capability. However, the principles of each type of equipment, as applied to creating effective strength gains, remains similar.)
- Elastic resistance cable or tubing (Elastic resistance can be classified as a cable system and can be used without pulleys or directed through pulleys. It can be attached to the wall or a door frame and provides unlimited and versatile exercise options. This stuff really works if you get pieces of tubing that are strong enough to effectively resist the exercise movement!)
- Training without equipment (Calisthenics and your own body weight have limitations with regard to progressive overload and working out at the right level of resistance.)

Choose strength equipment that offers you the option to increase resistance as you get stronger. Free weights, multistation weight machines, pulley/cable systems, and elastic resistance cables and tubing are good examples of equipment that can provide progressive overload. This type of equipment allows you to increase weight once you can perform more repetitions than your recommended range. This keeps you progressing and keeps the results coming.

Free Weights

Barbells and dumbbells generally have free weights or weight plates attached to them. Barbells are long, straight bars that allow you to attach weight plates to each end of the bar. When loaded, you need two hands to lift them, unless you're Rambo. Dumbbells are short bars with weight plates on both ends. Usually you lift one with each hand or use a single dumbbell in both hands, depending on the exercise. The plates can be attached securely with retaining collars or more permanent fixtures that eliminate the possibility of the free weight falling off during exercise.

Free weights are great because they don't take up much room, are inexpensive and versatile compared to machines, and offer numerous exercises that are biomechanically correct. You don't need $100,000 worth of equipment to get a great strength workout, yet you can replicate $100,000 worth of exercises with them!

Free weights work with your body, not against it, if you've been instructed correctly with regard to technique and you're using the right exercises. Free weights also require balance, stabilization, and coordination. That's important because what you do in everyday life, and the sports you participate in, also require balance, stabilization, and coordination.

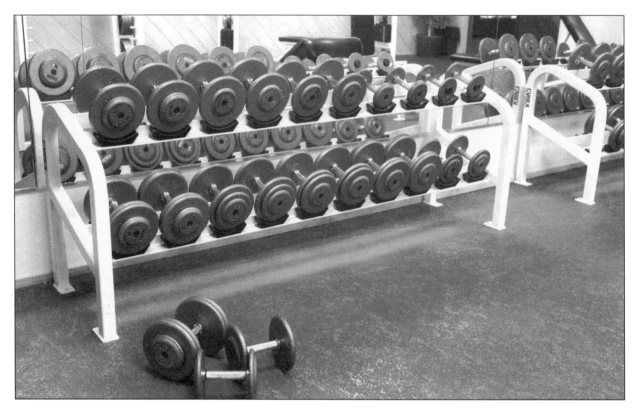

Figure 3.1 Fixed dumbbells.

Free-weight workouts don't take much time if you avoid adjustable dumbbells that require you to slide weight plates on and off and then secure them with safety collars so they don't slide onto your pretty face! Instead, go for fixed dumbbells. These are not adjustable and are bombproof with minimal maintenance. They don't come apart on you! You grab the pair you need, do your exercise, and you're on to the next one.

One very effective system I have seen on the market, with regard to cost and space efficiency, is the PowerBlock dumbbell system. The PowerBlock gives you a whole set of dumbbells in your home at minimal cost, and its unique design doesn't require much space. It's nice to have this versatility without taking up the space of an entire wall, which is required of a dumbbell rack that houses 10 to 15 pairs of dumbbells. Three sets are available which go up to 45, 90, and 120 pounds, and you can change from 5 pounds to 120 pounds in seconds.

When using free weights:

- Keep your concentration and focus.
- Lift weight that you can control.
- If the weight is hard to balance or control because it's too heavy or you've reached a point of fatigue, lower the weight and start again with less weight.
- Remove the weight carefully from the rack and replace it with precision and control back on to its stand. (Many injuries during strength training come from carelessly picking up or returning weight to storage racks, or the floor!)
- Learn how to move into and out of an exercise safely.

Multistation Weight Machines

Many home multistation strength gyms require you to push, pull, or curl in a predetermined range. (Some companies are now making commercial-quality equipment that allows the user to define the range of motion. This is trickling down to home-gym designs that allow greater biomechanical adjustability to some degree.) You've probably experienced a machine that doesn't feel right or creates discomfort in a joint. You could be performing an ineffective or unsafe exercise with no option to modify it. Before you buy, try out the machine and each exercise it offers. The range of motion should feel natural and comfortable, and at no point during a movement should you feel joint discomfort or pain. Additionally, many multistation gyms do not have many exercise options. Make sure you can target all the major muscle groups. Don't trust that all manufacturers know what they're doing and have your best interest placed first with regard to exercise design and selection. Often, they don't!

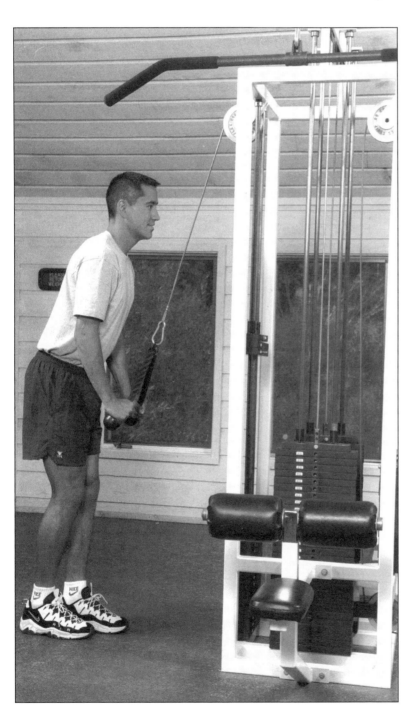

If you choose to purchase a higher-end home gym, you'll find it has multiple weight stacks, has a removable bench that lies flat and inclines at several different angles, and it can train most, if not all, of the major muscle groups. Plus, you can push yourself without needing a partner to spot you since the weight can't fall on you and it can take up as little as four by eight feet of space. (Check to make sure your ceiling height accommodates the machine.) Multiple weight stacks require fewer adjustments and cable connections as you move from exercise to exercise, and more than one person can work out at a time. The guide rods and cables will operate smoothly and quietly.

Figure 3.2   Multistation weight machine.

KEY POINT

Adding a full range of dumbbells to your workout arsenal will add all the strength exercise options you'll ever need, and you can use the bench that comes with the multistation gym.

Weight machines usually come with a stack of weights, although there are other effective options (e.g., Bowflex and the composite resistance rods provide comparable resistance, and they're easy to move since you don't have to cart around stacks of steel). When using stacked plates or selectorized plates, you select the amount of weight you want by inserting a T-shaped pin through a small hole drilled in each weight plate.

As we have discussed, one problem with machines is that they're usually designed as "one size fits all." You've heard that promise before and know what it gets you. Most machines use a cam design to alter the amount of weight you work against at different points through the range of motion. This represents a strength curve and what is called variable resistance. Do you think your strength curve is the same as the man or woman next to you who has arms the size of your legs? Do you believe for a minute your hips are the same width as your next-door neighbor, your arms and upper torso are of similar length to every person in the gym, and your strength is the same as the hulk wanting to take over the machine you're on? One size fits all just doesn't deliver much, to anyone!

Realize that weight machines won't fit everybody perfectly. If it feels wrong, don't use the machine. You may adjust until you're blue in the face and it'll never be right.

Do strength machines work? You betcha. They get similar results as tubing and free weights, when proper load is used. Results are not dependent on what type of equipment is being used or whether it's variable resistance. What counts is whether you're working to fatigue, generally between 6 and 20 reps.

Are multistation gyms really safer than other equipment? Maybe and maybe not! You always hear they're ideal for beginners because they're so safe, meaning the weight can't fall on you. Yet, I can already hear fingers crunching, hair stuck in pulley/cable systems ripping, and joints aching because people have been led to believe machines are perfectly safe. Be careful when you're around a weight stack. And although weight may never fall on you, if you fatigue quicker than you planned, you can surely have your upper limbs ripped from their attachments at the shoulder if you cannot control the weight back to its starting place. For example, a pullover exercise can turn into a nightmare called "super-stretch." If you did not take your Gumby-the-stretch-man pills that day, you could be crawling over to a phone and dialing 911.

Machines tend to isolate musculature. They don't require the kind of balance and stabilization needed for everyday activity and sports movement. So think about a balanced approach here. If you always train on machines, add some upper body dumbbell exercises, squats, and lunges to your routine.

And finally, machines generally are not portable (ever try to fit one in your suitcase?), and they are pricey. It's important to know how to work out with minimal equipment— such as free weights, dumbbells, and tubing— and still optimize your training results. This is especially true if you travel a lot. You never know what will be available to you when you're traveling, and this knowledge keeps you from missing a workout and losing hard-won fitness gains!

Elastic Resistance

I know what you're thinking: Aagh, come on—tubing? Let's get real and move to the machines and weight! Okay, I know I'm talking about sophisticated rubber bands, but do they ever work well. You can get them in different thicknesses to let you work harder, some have rotating handles which make them easier to use, they can travel with you, they take up little space, they're inexpensive, and they're effective! And, they're like free weights in that you can work with your body because the range of motion is not predetermined and they require some balance as you stretch the tube. You can easily hook them to your door (with a door attachment strap), which makes tubing even more versatile, and you can copy all of the same exercises you could do on a fancy $100,000 lineup of weight machines!

In other words, you have hundreds of exercises to choose from. If you work against a heavy enough resistance as provided by the tube thickness or by shortening the tube before you perform an exercise, you'll get the same results you would from weight machines or dumbbells.

> ### KEY POINT
>
> Muscles only know fatigue and correct mechanics; they cannot differentiate the type of equipment being used. Strength results are determined by working at sufficient exercise load or intensity.

a

b

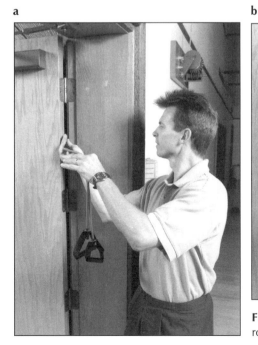
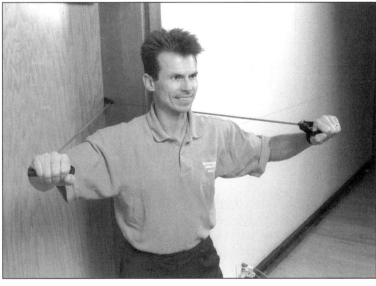

Figure 3.3 *(a)* Door attachment strap. *(b)* Tubing attached to door with rotating handles.

Calisthenics and Lifting Your Own Body Weight

The biggest drawback to using your body weight for strength exercises is that usually the exercise is too hard or too easy. And, if the amount of effort is just right, it's not long before it becomes too easy. Take push-ups or chin-ups as examples. Some people can't do any, others a straining few, and a small number can crank out reps until the cows come home. If the exercise is too hard or too easy, you're probably wasting your time.

Calisthenics and using body weight is not an issue of good or bad. Simply realize their limitations. You can use these types of exercises to maintain some level of strength, and a quick set of push-ups never hurt anyone. To determine their effectiveness, ask this question: can I fatigue the muscles I'm using in 6 to 20 reps? If you can't, you're not optimizing strength results or the use of your time!

EQUIPMENT ESSENTIALS: THE FINAL WORD

Don't believe all the gym stories that attest to a particular piece of equipment's overstated magnificence, effectiveness, and magical qualities. You've got to use the right equipment (defined by your goal), like using it, and use it correctly!

KEY POINT

How you use equipment—regardless of its cost or lack thereof—is of utmost importance. Having said that, running a close second, with regard to importance, is the quality of the equipment. Good technique can be short-circuited by equipment that doesn't even have good resale value when presented to a scrap metal reclamation yard!

Technically, and from a physiological standpoint, how the body adapts to overload it is not accustomed to (called the training effect) does not change. Neither does the body differentiate between one piece of equipment and the next. As pointed out earlier, the body only understands effective training and correct overload, regardless of equipment choice.

You need to ask the question, can the equipment I'm using deliver? In other words, principles of overload do not change. If the equipment allows you to exercise harder than your body is used to, and you enjoy doing it on a regular basis, you'll get results. On the other hand, high-priced equipment won't do the work for you or necessarily give you better results than less expensive equipment. However, you need to find a balance between useless equipment and high-grade (not necessarily top-dollar) home gym exercise equipment. Obviously, it is you, following the right training guidelines and using correct exercise technique, that optimizes result.

The key is to select equipment that can meet the overload and biomechanical standards described in this book, and you don't need to have an unlimited budget to purchase equipment that gets it done. On the other hand, if all the extra gadgets and creature comforts of top-of-the-line models motivate you to exercise and budget is not of concern, then they're worth the price.

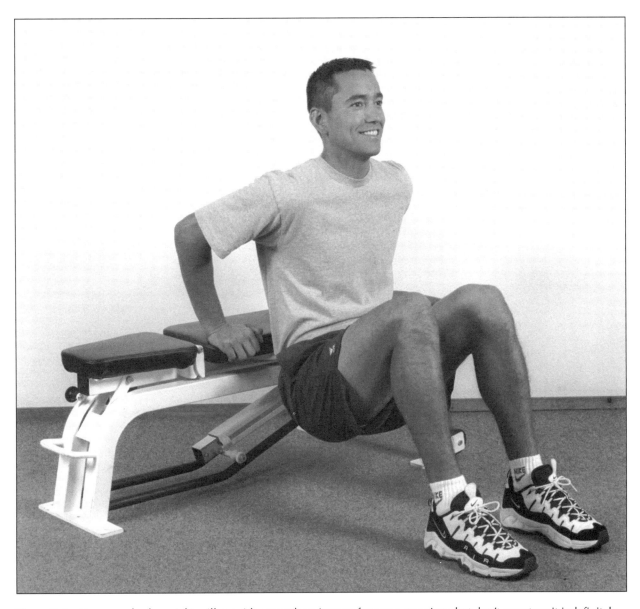

Figure 3.4   Your own body weight will provide enough resistance for some exercises, but don't count on it indefinitely.

Besides the time-tested cardio machines and strength training equipment already discussed, several pieces of exercise apparatus are incredibly productive in contributing to a well-rounded, interesting, versatile, and effective training program. In fact, many of these options are some of the best kept secrets in the fitness industry!

Following are equipment choices that are some combination of inexpensive (or at least cost effective when compared to the options), portable, and versatile. Some of the options are great to use even in an atmosphere in which there is a wide assortment of equipment, such as a commercial club. None of them compromises the workout. Even in situations in which you have every equipment option, you might want to return to these choices because they provide fun and effective variety if your mind and body are tired of the same workout.

Cost Effective, Versatile, and Portable Equipment Options

1. Dumbbells

   a. The PowerBlock dumbbell system allows you to strength train safely and effectively in your home with unlimited exercise variety, minimal space requirements, and minimal dollar investment.

   b. An alternative is several pairs of fixed (the weight plates are secured in a "bombproof" manner) dumbbells that are appropriate to your current strength level.

   c. Changeable (nonfixed) dumbbells are another OK choice, but be aware of safety issues. Secure the quick-release locking collars before every exercise and never hold them over your face.

   d. PlateMates are the perfect way to add microincrements of $1\frac{1}{4}$, $2\frac{1}{2}$, $3\frac{3}{4}$ and 5 pounds to your exslting dumbbells or multigym weight stack. This helps you avoid the dangerous alternative of large jumps in weight, for example, a minimum of 5 to 10 pound increments. You simply add the magnetic PlateMate onto a fixed-weight dumbbell or weight stack. They are available in $1\frac{1}{4}$ and $2\frac{1}{2}$ pound sizes (combine them to get the $3\frac{3}{4}$ and 5 pound increases). And don't worry, they are very secure!

2. Multistation and pulley/cable systems

   Some strength training systems allow you to strength train safely and effectively in your home with unlimited exercise variety, minimal space requirements, and reasonable dollar investment! The Bowflex system, for example, is a pulley/cable system that uses composite rods for progressive resistance and is a great choice for a multistation gym if you don't like the idea of weight stacks and restricted movement patterns. Test the Bowflex (it is not for everyone) and other multistation units before you buy!

3. Elastic resistance

   Elastic resistance devices such as tubing or bands provide variable resistance with many different strengths of tubing. Attached handles and bars make it easy to perform a variety of exercises. Door attachments and wall-mounted units increase elastic resistance versatility.

4. Stability ball

   This air-filled ball is used extensively by physical therapists to strengthen and stretch the body. It is especially well suited for strengthening the abdominal and back areas, provides a cushion of air to work from, supports your body, and you can change how hard you work by how you position your body on the ball (i.e., the stability ball can provide progressive resistance overload by adjusting body position). Once you've trained on the ball, you'll never go back to traditional floor exercises. The stability ball provides major muscle group overload and flexibility training. It can also be used as an exercise bench.

5. Partner-assisted manual resistance

   Partner-assisted resistance is a very effective method that allows an increase in overload and assistance with range of motion and correct technique. Obviously, you need a trusted and knowledgeable workout companion to use partner resistance.

6. Body weight as resistance

   A variety of exercise positions, such as a push-ups or heel raises, comprise this technique. Limitations of using this type of resistance were mentioned in the section on calisthenic exercise.

7. Adjustable step platform

   An adjustable step platform can be used for cardio and strength training in combination with weight or tubing. It doubles as a flat, incline, or decline strength bench.

8. Adjustable exercise bench

   This piece of equipment replaces the need for two benches because it is adjustable from flat to vertical. You can use it to perform many exercises from standing or seated positions.

9. Manual rowing machine (nonflywheel)

   A manual rowing machine can be used for cardio or strength training by changing resistance. Quick fatigue (30 to 90 seconds) and more resistance will result in strength gains, whereas high repetition overload (three minutes or longer) offers cardiovascular training outcomes. By facing forward on the seat and pushing, you can work the triceps, front of the shoulder, and chest. Face backward and pull and you target the biceps, back of the shoulders, and the upper back.

Quick Index:

PART II

Your Training Components

4 Optimize Your Flexibility

Flexibility training is probably one of the most overlooked, poorly executed, poorly understood, and undervalued components of physical fitness and overall personal health. Yet achieving and maintaining flexibility is an important factor in reaching your optimal health and performance potential.

Why stretch? Has your running stride turned into a shuffle or do you feel stiff and move jerkily? Stretching lets you move your joints easily. Stretching all of the main muscle groups leads to muscle balance (i.e., some muscles won't be tighter than others). Because supple and mobile joints move easily through a range of motion and require less effort to do so, you'll be less likely to injure a muscle, and you can improve your performance.

Improved flexibility also leads to good posture. Tight neck, shoulder, and chest muscles lead to a rounded back and head position that is tilted forward and up. Tightness in your hips and the back of your thighs can lead to a pelvis that doesn't move freely. Tight hip muscles can also cause your low back to become excessively arched. Sound uncomfortable? It is! This type of posture can lead to chronic, unrelenting neck or low back pain. A simple stretching routine done regularly requires little time and can reduce pain in your body and contribute to silky smooth, unrestricted movement. It should be a very enjoyable, relaxing part of your workout that you look forward to.

Flexibility is most simply defined as the range of motion available to a joint or joints. However, the joint's *normal* range of motion is not always healthy or adequate for your movement needs. Too much flexibility or overly restricted movement at the joints in the body can lead to problems.

Functional flexibility or functional range of motion is a relatively new concept that is gaining momentum. Accordingly, the goal of stretching changes from simply increasing range of motion to improving the flexibility necessary for a specific activity, sport, or daily chore—without compromising joint stability. (Overly mobile joints can lead to as many, if not more, problems than a general lack of flexibility!) This functional type of stretching can also be termed "usable" flexibility and represents the concept of functional range of motion.

You're probably looking to gain usable flexibility with minimal risk, discomfort, and time commitment. Extreme ranges of motion and contorted stretch postures are high risk for most people. But, smart stretching will yield favorable results, with minimal risk and time investment, and no pain.

BENEFITS OF STRETCHING

Too often, committed exercisers fail to slow down and pause before rushing off to their scheduled and busy days. However, by taking the time for flexibility training, you can give yourself a great opportunity to reflect on both short- and long-term accomplishments. Besides important physical benefits, stretching creates an opportunity to increase your sense of self-esteem by acknowledging what, for example, you have just accomplished during your most recent workout. Let's take a look at what improved flexibility can lead to.

Better posture

Improved posture can help you avoid chronic injuries due to poor postural alignment and muscular imbalances. Flexibility training can help realign skeletal structure that has adapted to habits of incorrect posture and poor exercise technique. You will find it easier to maintain proper posture throughout the day. Stretching can improve or maintain your appearance since it helps you keep or attain good posture.

> ### KEY POINT
> Having adequate flexibility in all of your major muscle groups will make the efforts of daily activities and sport performance less strenuous and more efficient.

Furthermore, there is strong scientific evidence that the risk of incurring low back pain and experiencing stress to the lumbar spine (low back) can be avoided with increased pelvic mobility.

You need sufficient flexibility *and* strength in the hamstrings, gluteus minimus and medius (muscles of the outer hip area), gluteus maximus (buttocks muscle), hip flexors (front of the hips), and low back musculature.

Increased Range of Motion

Increased range of motion available at a joint or joints can provide for greater ease of movement and result in safer and more effective movement. A mobile joint moves more easily through a range of motion, requires less energy, and feels better.

Development of Functional Flexibility

The development of functional, or usable, flexibility entails challenging range of motion and balance in a manner that prepares you for daily activities. Functional movement in daily activities and sport skills is often dynamic in nature. Righting yourself after losing your balance or standing on one leg are good examples of the requirements of dynamic movement. You'll discover that many of the stretches found at the end of this chapter challenge balance while you stretch.

Injury Prevention

Most experts agree that stretching correctly reduces the likelihood of injury. A good stretching program makes it easier to stretch muscle tissue and increases the range of motion available to the muscle tissue, making it less likely that a stretching force could cause an injury. Because of this, you are less likely to incur injury because the maximum range (called the elastic limit) available to the muscle tissue before damage occurs will not likely, or as easily, be exceeded.

Increased Blood Supply, Nutrients, and Joint Synovial Fluid

Alternately holding and releasing sustained stretches increases tissue temperature (along with an adequate warm-up), circulation, and nutrient delivery through the blood. Regular stretching decreases the viscosity or thickness of synovial fluid present in the joints of the body, which enables nutrients to be transported more readily to cartilage that covers the surfaces of the bones that come into contact with one another. This change in qualitative aspects of synovial joint fluid may lead to a decrease in degenerative joint diseases (i.e., arthritis or osteoarthritis) and allow more freedom of movement at the joint.

> **KEY POINT**
>
> Think of stretching as a free lube job. You'll enjoy the feeling of greased joints!

Reduced Muscle Soreness

Although stretching cannot correct the consequences of exercise that results in an injured muscle or connective tissue, research indicates that slow, static stretching performed after exercise reduces or prevents delayed muscular soreness and enhances recovery from exercise. Although the physiologic reason for this effect is far from clear, it may be partially attributed to the increase in muscle temperature, circulation, enhanced blood supply, and nutrient delivery from the alternating tension and release experienced in the muscles during stretching activity.

Personal Enjoyment, Relaxation, and Reduced Stress

When conducted in the proper environment and with correct technique, stretching encourages muscular as well as mental relaxation. Subjective, personal enjoyment and physical release through stretching can lead to a reduction in overall stress levels. In addition, alternating tension and release on the muscle during stretching promotes optimal nutrition to the muscle, may decrease the accumulation of toxins in the muscles, and reduces the likelihood of adaptive shortening or decreased flexibility in the muscle.

ANATOMY AND TYPES OF STRETCH

It's important to understand what connective tissues are being affected by stretching, what the mechanical characteristics of the tissues are (is the tissue easy or hard to stretch and under what circumstances?), what you're actually targeting when you're stretching (by the way, it isn't the muscle!), and what the different types of stretching are.

Flexibility is influenced by a variety of factors, some of which may be changed, while others are unable to be altered, or if altered could lead to injury. These include the following:

- Genetic inheritance (don't worry about this one; everyone can improve 100 percent from their starting point).
- Joint structure itself (by design, joints restrict movement to some degree so that you will not flop around like a rag doll).
- Tension (partial contraction) in the muscle (get rid of this by stretching in a warm environment, without bouncing).
- Connective tissue limitations within the muscles (this is what you're really stretching once you get the muscle to relax).
- Tendons (they have to be rigid to transmit the forces of muscle contraction to the bones so that you can move efficiently).
- Ligaments (they stabilize joints).
- Skin surrounding the joint (this has very little influence).
- Neuromuscular influences (sensory organs such as the muscle spindle and Golgi tendon organ can enhance or inhibit stretching results).

Anatomy of Stretch

Connective tissues of the joint include cartilage, ligaments, tendons, and muscle fascia. Cartilage is often present between bones to provide a degree of protection for bone surfaces that come into contact with one another, by providing padding and shock-absorbing capabilities. The fibers in cartilage are more stretchable or forgiving. This characteristic enhances its shock-absorbing capability without increasing the risk of tearing.

Ligaments connect bone to bone and offer stability and integrity to joint structures in areas of the body such as the spine, knee, and shoulder. Tendons connect muscles to bone. The force of muscle contraction is transferred via the tendinous attachment of the muscles to the skeletal system. This results in efficient bodily movement.

Three layers of muscle fascia wrap the muscle. Endomysium (pronounced "en-do-MISS-ee-um") wraps individual muscle fibers or cells. The perimysium wraps groups or bundles of muscle fibers, and the epimysium wraps the entire muscle. These various layers of fascia culminate in the tendons of the muscle.

The muscle and its fascial layers look somewhat like a twist-tied piece of candy. The candy represents the muscle; the paper wrappings represent muscle fascia; and the ends of the candy, where the paper is twisted, represent tendons that attach the muscle to bone. (It should be noted that neither the muscle's tendons or fibers are actually twisted.) This image offers a good way for you to visualize the physical look of the muscle and connective tissue arrangement (see figure 4.17). Stay with me—we're going somewhere with this information!

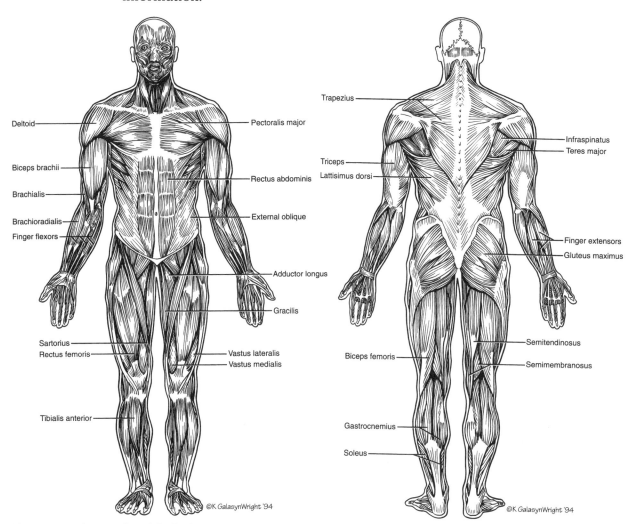

Figure 4.1 The muscles of the body.

What Is Being Stretched During Flexibility Training?

Now that you've got the picture, here's a key fact. Since muscle fascia is easy and desirable to stretch when compared to ligaments and tendons, this makes it the most significant, changeable, limiting factor for gains in flexibility. In other words, if your muscles are relaxed (absent of tension) when you stretch, what accounts for a change in range of motion is your ability to stretch fascia, not muscle! You don't want to stretch ligaments or tendons or strain muscle fibers, because you'll end up with an injury. Muscle fascia accounts for almost 50 percent of the resistance to stretch or range of motion at a given joint, and it's easy to stretch.

Muscle itself can be stretched to 150 percent of its length if relaxed and unrestricted by muscle fascia. For example, a muscle in its relaxed state of 10 inches in length could be stretched to 15 inches of length abruptly with no injurious effects. (It should be noted that muscle begins to break down if the muscle is stretched beyond 160 percent of its normal length. More is not better!)

> ## KEY POINT
> Muscle fascia gives muscle the ability to change length. An effective stretching program depends on your ability to stretch muscle fascia.

It's simple. Here's several years of cellular physiology packed into a few sentences. Ligaments and tendons are hard to stretch because of the roles they play in stabilization and muscle force production. Muscle fascia is easy to stretch. Liken muscle fascia to candy taffy. When taffy is cold, it is brittle and breakable. Try to bend cold taffy and it shatters. On the other hand, when taffy is warm, it stretches. That's why you warm up; when your body is cold, the muscle fascia is far less pliable. If you stretch the taffy (muscle fascia) gradually into a newly lengthened position, it will cool and adapt to this new position. Over time, the change will be permanent. The risk of injury while stretching is close to nonexistent if you warm up and don't bounce. That's called smart stretching!

How the Nervous System Influences Stretching Results

Here's a little more science. Two sensory organs, the muscle spindle and the Golgi tendon organ (GTO), have implications for flexibility training. If you don't take advantage of them, you're likely to get injured or won't see the results you'd like. Understanding this aspect of neuroanatomy will help you trust the recommendations under the section that details how to stretch.

The muscle spindles are located between muscle fibers. They measure changes in the resting length of the muscle, changes that occur in the length of the muscle during activity, and the speed at which lengthening occurs. This information that the muscle spindle sensory organ picks up is sent via the nerves back to the brain for processing. Muscle spindles help the body maintain muscle tone and good posture—your head jerks back to an upright posture when you're groggy, or you can feel the muscles in your lower leg alternately contract and relax if you stand in one place for a while. And spindles present a defense mechanism, through the stretch reflex, that can help prevent muscle injury.

If your muscles are stretched too fast, the spindles initiate the stretch reflex. (The stretch reflex is also referred to as the myotatic stretch reflex. This is important to know only if you like to practice your Greek or impress your friends.) This reflex causes the muscle group that is being stretched too fast, as interpreted by the muscle spindle, to automatically shorten and protect itself from being overstretched or injured.

If you try to lengthen muscle fascia (commonly referred to as stretching) while the muscle itself is contracting, the risk of injury to the muscle is obvious. The resultant situation finds the muscle shortening while you are trying to lengthen it. Since the force produced by the stretch reflex is proportional to the force or speed of the stretch, if you stretch in a slow and controlled fashion, the stretch reflex may be avoided or be of low intensity.

KEY POINT

To avoid the stretch reflex, stretch without bouncing and with control. Ease into your stretches.

The Golgi tendon organ (GTO)—this is that other sensory organ you're going to exploit—is located in the muscle tendon where tendons attach muscle to bone. GTOs are sensitive to muscle force production and monitor tension in the muscle. When their force thresholds are exceeded, their response causes the affected muscles to relax, which is the opposite effect of the muscle spindle (remember, it causes the muscle to shorten). This GTO response is referred to as an inverse stretch reflex or inverse myotatic reflex (there's another one of those terms). The GTOs' signal to relax overrides the muscle spindles' signal to contract. This in turn relaxes the muscle group you're stretching. Remember, a relaxed muscle allows you to target the muscle fascia and helps you avoid injuring your muscles. Your goal during stretching is to relax the muscle, "fire" the GTOs, and avoid activating the muscle spindle.

KEY POINT

Stretching right involves using the responses of the muscle spindle and GTOs to your advantage. Now you begin to understand that a base of knowledge exists that supports and directs you to a best way to stretch.

The final nervous system response you can use to improve your stretching result is called reciprocal innervation. When a muscle group contracts (the agonist), its opposing or antagonistic muscle group automatically relaxes. Reciprocal innervation is a technique that you should use when you stretch, and, best of all, you don't have to think. It is true—some stuff just happens!

For example, if the goal is to stretch the hamstring group (back of the thigh) from a supine (on your back) position, tightening the quadriceps (against) or straightening the leg at the knee would cause the hamstrings muscle (antagonist) to relax because of reciprocal innervation. In general motor movement, reciprocal innervation is important because it allows for the occurrence of coordinated motor movement. Have you ever tried to run forward, but the muscles on the opposite side of your body pull you backward? During stretching, reciprocal innervation is a reflex mechanism that can be taken advantage of to create a relaxed muscle. Potentially, this will allow for more effective stretching to take place.

As you will see, the best stretching takes advantage of muscle spindles, GTOs, and reciprocal innervation to promote muscle relaxation and optimal stretching conditions that will increase your flexibility—and it's easy!

Types of Stretch

Forces responsible for stretch can be broadly categorized as either active or passive. An active stretch occurs when an agonist muscle (or prime mover) moves a body part through a range of motion, and the force provided by the active contraction of the muscle stretches the opposing (antagonist) muscles. For example, if the elbow is flexed (bent), the contracting biceps actively stretch the opposing or triceps (back of the upper arm) musculature.

Passive stretches occur when outside forces assist in the stretching process. Gravity, momentum or motion, a trainer or workout partner applying passive force to a body part, or an assisting force provided by some part of your own body (e.g., pulling your leg forward into a hamstrings stretch from a position on your back) are examples of passive forces that can help you increase flexibility.

KEY POINT

Optimal stretching will combine active and passive stretching.

How Flexibility Is Gained

Two basic categories identify how flexibility is gained. Static flexibility generally refers to a combination of active and passive movements that lengthen the muscles and fascia in a *controlled* manner. Once lengthened, the position is sustained (held without bouncing) for about 10 to 60 seconds.

Dynamic (or ballistic) flexibility involves the use of momentum to gain an advantage in "overstretching" an area of the body. This is traditionally referred to as ballistic stretching. Although there may be sufficient reasoning to justify this type of stretching in elite athletic participation, the risk versus effectiveness should be carefully examined with regard to your program goals.

A professional tennis player needs sufficient dynamic flexibility in the shoulder to slam a tennis serve 120-plus mph. Likewise, a recreational exerciser and mother needs sufficient dynamic flexibility in various joints of the body to play softball on the weekends and care for her children. Normal range of motion attained through static-controlled stretching will be sufficient to meet the dynamic needs of mom, whereas dynamic flexibility training might be required to meet the demands imposed on the body of a professional tennis player.

Many researchers conclude that the use of ballistic flexibility is probably important in explosive events. This includes sports and activities such as gymnastics, sprinting, some types of dance, and diving. This simply recognizes that ballistic movements are contained in these sports and does not support ballistic stretching as a safe and effective way to stretch for the majority of the population.

In fact, many experts suggest that abrupt stretching may lead to injury. That is why most fitness experts generally recommend static stretching programs that gradually increase range of motion, and hold stretching positions with static force (no bouncing) applied during the stretch.

PNF Stretching

Since we're talking about high-risk stretching procedures, PNF needs to be addressed. Proprioceptive neuromuscular facilitation (PNF) stretching is a technique that can provide significant gains in flexibility, which is why PNF stretching is very popular with athletes whose events require above-average flexibility.

PNF stretching requires the muscle to be "put on" a maximal stretch, then contracted maximally for several seconds using an isometric contraction (no movement occurs at the joint being stretched). Afterwards, active and/or passive stretch techniques are applied to attempt to further increase range of motion. PNF stretching puts you at an increased risk for injury simply because the muscle is stretched maximally and then is required to produce a maximal force in this vulnerable position. In theory, this maximal stretch and force production fires the GTO and relaxes the muscle, which can lead to more effective stretching. (The GTO can also be fired with sufficiently intense, sustained, and static stretching!) No doubt about it, PNF stretching is an advanced form of flexibility training.

It cannot be overemphasized that more aggressive attempts to increase flexibility (such as PNF stretching) should be met with careful scrutiny. The risk of injury can greatly increase, while the gains in flexibility you receive will often be about the same as those gained when using sustained, static stretching.

Type of Stretching That Works Best

As discussed, the major limiting factor affecting flexibility is muscle fascia, and almost half of the resistance to range of motion is related to your ability to effectively stretch muscle fascia. This is a factor that can be modified without negatively affecting joint stability and creating an increased risk for injury.

KEY POINT

When deciding what technique or combination of stretching techniques to use, look to science first, then balance this factual information with your individual makeup and goals, and evaluate the risk involved with each approach when compared to the potential result.

Static stretching gains the most support in terms of safety and effectiveness. The amount of muscle fascia lengthening that remains after the stretching force is removed is greatest when using low-force, long-duration (10- to 60-second) static stretches. Static stretching offers a low incidence of injury potential. If your goal is to attain functional flexibility, this can easily and effectively be attained with static stretching.

Ballistic stretching involves the use of momentum to gain an advantage in "overstretching" an area of the body. Arguments *against* ballistic stretching include the following:

- Increased muscle soreness.
- Lack of tissue adaptation. Tissue adaptation is time dependent. Ballistic stretching does not allow for a lengthened position of the fascia to be sustained.
- Initiation of the stretch reflex and an increase in muscular tension.
- Decreased neurological adaptations, especially the muscle spindle and its time-dependent threshold. If the goal is to reset the muscle spindle to a higher level, meaning it won't fire as easily and cause tension in the muscle, ballistic stretching is not the right choice.

Experts in the field disagree with the popular notion that PNF stretching in its various forms yields far greater results than standard static stretching. When you read that one method is the best, you need to ask, for whom and for what? If attaining functional flexibility is the goal, PNF stretching might be inappropriate given its associated risks.

BROOKS'S BEST WAY TO STRETCH

To review, several things determine if the stretch you're doing is helpful or harmful. They include

- the type of force, whether active, passive, static, or ballistic;
- the use of correct technique during the stretch and exercise position;
- the duration of the stretch (10 to 60 seconds);
- the intensity of the stretch (it needs to be comfortably-uncomfortable or to the point of mild tension); and
- the temperature of the muscle (it needs to be warm) during the stretch.

If the muscles are stretched too fast or ballistically, muscle spindles initiate a stretch reflex, which causes the affected muscle group to automatically shorten and protect it from being overstretched and injured. The resultant increase in muscle tension hinders the stretching process and can lead to injury. If the stretch is performed slowly with control, the stretch reflex may be avoided or be of low intensity. Yet, if the static stretch is of sufficient intensity, you can cause the GTOs to fire, which will help relax the targeted muscles causing your stretching to be more effective.

Remember, many of the gains in any fitness component are often related to your effort, focus, concentration, and consistency in the effort, as well as the correctness of the approach. This certainly holds true for flexibility training.

Warm Up Before You Stretch

Remember, muscle fascia's physical properties are not unlike those of candy taffy. When it is warm, it is stretchable. When it is cold (the body is not warmed up), it is unbending. Because of these physical characteristics, you should warm the body first and hold sustained stretches so that the muscle fascia can literally cool in a new and lengthened position. This representation should help you better understand the goals of your stretching program and help you visualize what happens when you stretch.

Flexibility training should be preceded by at least three to five minutes of warm-up activity that allows you to move through an easy range of motion and never beyond a point of gentle tension or strain. Keep your movements fluid, rhythmic, and controlled. Three to five minutes of slow walking, jogging, biking, or rowing are good examples.

If the goal is to concentrate on flexibility gains, it's a good idea to do so only after an extensive warm-up (15 to 20 minutes), or after warming up and participating in your chosen activity. Then, focus your stretching efforts after the cool-down.

Stretching is not a good warm-up. You've seen joggers gather curbside in the morning to stretch their calves to warm up. Forcing range of motion when muscles are cold is less effective at increasing range of motion safely and can cause injury.

KEY POINT

Stretching may take place any time after you've adequately warmed up. Stretching is different from warming up. Warm up to warm up and stretch to stretch!

A flexibility warm-up and cool-down can be defined as stretching that is participated in before or after an activity to improve performance, reduce the risk of injury, or enhance recovery. The goal is *not* to increase range of motion, but to prepare your body for upcoming activity or to facilitate recovery from activity.

Flexibility training is defined as a planned, deliberate, progressive, and regular program of stretching that causes permanent (plastic) elongation of muscle fascia without causing, or contributing to, injury. Flexibility training's focus is to aggressively pursue increases in range of motion available at the joint, or joints, being stretched.

Stretching Right

I use a combination of active, controlled passive, and static stretching technique with my clients.

Step 1: To use this method, an active contraction is initiated with agonist muscles. For example, stand or sit. Hold your arm out in front of you and parallel to the ground. Draw your arm across the body as far as you can without momentum and with no outside assistance. (This invokes the nervous system

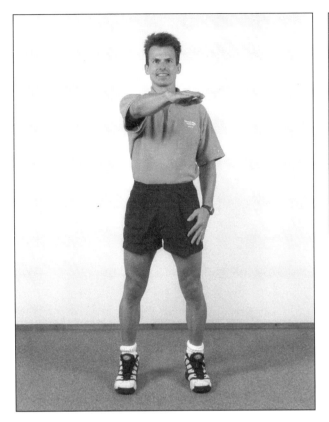

Figure 4.2   Here's an example of active contraction: from a standing or sitting position, hold your arm out in front of you and parallel to the ground. Draw your arm across the body as far as you can without momentum and with no outside assistance.

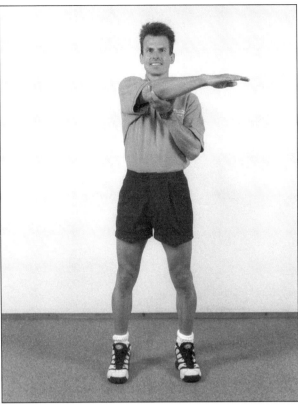

Figure 4.3   Assisted contraction uses outside force to assist in the stretch. This time, use the hand opposite of the arm being stretched to gently, and in a controlled manner, pull the arm a little further across the body.

reflex called reciprocal innervation and causes the antagonist muscle(s) on the opposite side to relax.)

This begins the stretch process and defines your active range of motion. Once active range of motion is determined or set, you have a better idea of a safe range of movement for that particular joint and muscle group(s).

Step 2: Step 1 is followed by an application of an outside or passive force that is used to enhance movement through a greater range of motion. For example, use the hand opposite the arm being stretched to gently, and in a controlled manner, pull the arm a little farther across the body. The tension felt in the back of the shoulder should be tolerable and sustainable (see figure 4.3).

Step 3: Finally, a static and sustained stretch is held for about 10 to 60 seconds while you maintain the application of the passive, outside assistance of your hand on the arm being stretched.

Use these three steps as you perform each of the 15 stretches found at the end of this chapter.

Following are basic guidelines to follow for safe and effective flexibility improvement:

- Always wear clothing that is comfortable, loose, and not restrictive. You want to stretch your muscle tissue, not the fabric in your jeans!

- Stretch all of the major muscle groups of the body for balance and bodily symmetry, because flexibility is specific to each joint. But, concentrate on the areas of the body that generally lack adequate flexibility. These include the chest, front of the shoulder, front of the hips (hip flexors), back of the upper legs (hamstrings), and the back of the lower legs (calves).

- Always find a body position that is comfortable for you. If the exercise is uncomfortable, select an alternative variation that stretches the same muscle groups, or modify the stretch. Your goal is to effectively stretch your muscle tissue, not to assume a twisted posture that is unbearable and may hurt you.

- Perform static stretching after a thorough warm-up of at least three to five minutes. This increases body and muscle temperature, and the likelihood that good gains in range of motion will be attained.

- Hold stretches for about 10 to 60 seconds. Holding stretches longer than a minute can increase the risk of injury.

- Hold each stretch at the point of mild tension or tightness. This represents exercise intensity. Stretch to the point at which movement or range of motion is limited at the joint. Stretching to an intensity that could be described as "comfortably uncomfortable" is OK if the stretch can be sustained. Do not stretch to the point of pain. You're stretching too hard if your muscles begin to feel like overtightened guitar strings that are ready to pop!

- The recommended frequency for stretching is a *minimum* of three times per week, although stretching daily is encouraged. A little bit done daily will take you a long way and help you avoid tightness.

- Perform one to four set(s) of a stretch or stretches per muscle group each time you stretch.

- Perform stretches after the muscle is relaxed and in a slow and controlled manner. Progress gradually to greater ranges of motion. When coming out of a stretch, release slowly.

- Breathe regularly throughout your stretches. You know you're not breathing if your eyes are about to explode from their sockets!

- Use subtle variations for given positions to stretch muscles in a variety of ways. The muscles of the body generally have various fiber direction alignments and orientations. By varying stretches, these structural arrangements within a given muscle, or muscles, will more likely be challenged. This may lead to overall greater flexibility improvement.

- Focus on proper stretching positions and techniques that do not put you at risk because of extreme or contorted postures.

- Design programming and assessment that measure improvement in flexibility. Assess and evaluate weaknesses and improvement in flexibility or areas of postural concern on an ongoing basis.

- Participate in a stretching program on a regular basis. Possibly the most important factor in stretching, after identifying and using correct stretching methods, is consistency and patience.

> **KEY POINT**
>
> Be sure to position yourself correctly (see Brooks's Top 15 Stretches, page 81) to maximize stretching gains and personal comfort and limit your chances of hurting yourself.

These guidelines are, of course, not fixed in stone. Recent research suggests that four sets of 15 to 20 seconds per stretch might result in *optimal* flexibility gains. However, the guidelines I have outlined can encompass a wide range of personal goals and available time commitments while still ensuring excellent flexibility gains.

WHEN TO STRETCH

When is the best time to fit stretching into your program? The answer, of course, is when it is most enjoyed and *accepted* by you. Some people don't like to take time for stretching that lasts more than a minute. If this matches your personality, sneak stretches in between resistance-training exercises as active recovery. If you look forward to the quiet time out, relaxation, and stress reduction that an extended series of stretches provides, then create a stretching program that gives you this break within your workouts.

Beyond this most important concept of what suits your personality and fits into your schedule, the optimal time to stretch also depends on your goals, the amount of warm-up that has taken place, and the type of activity you're going to participate in.

Gradual, low-level, rhythmic warm-up movement is essential prior to stretching. The warm-up activity should move through an easy range of motion, never going beyond a point perceived as excessive strain. The movements should be kept fluid, rhythmic, and controlled.

Duration of a warm-up depends on the activity being participated in and your individual preferences, based on personal experience. In other words, consider what works, but weigh it against what science indicates is optimal.

If stretches are performed during the warm-up preceding cardiovascular activity, the stretches should not last more than about 10 seconds and should be interspersed throughout the warm-up. In this case, the goal of the warm-up is to allow for a redistribution of blood to the working muscles in preparation for cardiovascular activity. Holds longer than 10 seconds may inhibit an effective blood shift to the muscles that are going to be used.

> **KEY POINT**
>
> To increase range of motion, it may be best to perform stretching after cardiovascular training because the muscle fascia will be very warm and more likely to respond to flexibility training.

Stretch During Strength Training

While it is a good idea to perform resistance training exercise through an active and full range of motion, this type of training *does not* replace flexibility training. Remember, active stretching during resistance training can be limited by the strength of the agonist (the muscle working) and/or lack of flexibility in the opposing muscle, which can interfere with the agonist's movement.

Sport-Specific Stretching

If you're going out for a leisurely, steady-rate run or walk, it may not be necessary—and in fact, may cause more harm—to stretch prior to the activity. If you start at a slow pace and gradually increase the pace, there is little risk for injury. No extreme ranges of motion or ballistic movement must be prepared for in this case, and stretching after the workout makes the most sense.

Try to match the flexibility exercises to the demands of the upcoming activity. As mentioned, extreme ranges of motion are not necessary prior to a fitness walking or running program to which you're accustomed. However, if you're going to perform a 5K race at your fastest walking or running pace, or participate in an aggressive match of singles tennis, a more thorough warm-up and stretching segment may better prepare you for the energy demands and range-of-motion and biomechanical stresses of high-intensity activity.

Competitive sports usually represent a different situation, too. A cross-country team might engage in a 10- or 15-minute run to warm the body. If the team is going to train with performance intervals, which demand all-out efforts and extreme range of motion when compared to steady-rate (easy) training, stretching is a prudent choice before interval training, but only after adequate warm-up. After initially stretching, the team may go for an additional jog of two or three miles, intersperse easy speed play (speed up and slow down) during the jog, perform the interval workout, cool down with a jog, and engage in stretching or flexibility training again postworkout. This approach is time intensive, yet very effective and appropriate for an athlete's commitment.

KEY POINT

Stretch . . . when you ache, when you're tense, in the morning, when you're stiff, when you're in a line, when you haven't moved in a while. Stretch and regularly fidget! It's good for you, feels great, keeps your body from getting used to poor posture, and keeps you aware of what your body is doing!

When *Not* to Stretch

Some situations in which it may not be best for you to stretch include the following:

- Within the first 24 to 72 hours following muscle or tendon trauma
- Following muscle strains and ligament sprains
- When joints or muscles are infected, inflamed, or hurt
- After a recent fracture

- When discomfort is present (Do not "work through" or "stretch out" painful areas.)
- When sharp pains are felt in the joint or muscle
- If osteoporosis exists or is suspected

Consult with the appropriate medical professional if you have questions. Rest and ice may be the simple solution in many of the instances cited. However, an expert and accurate professional opinion is necessary before proceeding.

BROOKS'S TOP 15 STRETCHES (AND HOW TO DO THEM)

Following are 15 stretches and lots of variations that target the muscles you use when, for example, you walk, hike, jog or run, cycle, strength train, or cross-train. These top stretches will meet your flexibility needs by targeting every major body area, especially those tight areas such as the back of the thighs and lower legs, front and outer part of the hip, chest, and front of the shoulder. Doing all 15 stretches will give you a full-body stretch that lengthens and relaxes the muscles that are working the hardest during your workouts and throughout your day.

You can perform this series of stretches all at once during your workout, do a stretch or two every few minutes during your workout for active recovery, or use them throughout your day. It's not necessary to perform every stretch during each of your workouts, nor is it important to lump all 15 stretches into a continuous time frame. Do what works! If you like interspersing your stretches throughout the workout, then do it. If you like the feel of a continuous stretch segment, then do it. Just don't leave out your stretching.

Be sure to hold each stretch for about 10 to 60 seconds. Don't bounce. You should feel a gentle stretch in the muscle. Avoid stretching to the point of pain. Position yourself comfortably, ease into each stretch, and breathe naturally. If you can't get the stretch to feel comfortable for your unique body type, even after modifying body position, don't use it. Try a variation or use another stretch that targets that same body part.

Quick Index:

stretch

1

Arm Pull-Back

Body Parts Targeted:
Front of the shoulders; chest

Muscles Stretched:
Anterior deltoid; pectoralis major

Execution of Stretch:
Stand with your feet shoulder-width apart, knees bent slightly, and toes pointing straight ahead. Let your arms hang relaxed to either side of your body. Expand the chest and pull your shoulders back by squeezing your shoulder blades toward each other. Slightly bend your elbows as you clasp your hands behind your back. Slowly straighten your arms as you lift your hands upward with control. Raise your hands until you feel mild tension in the shoulder/chest region. Lower your arms, then bend your elbows and release your hands from one another, with control.

Technique and Stretch Tips:
Don't bend over at the waist. You'll place unnecessary stress on your back and it doesn't make the stretch more effective. Keep your shoulders pulled back and avoid rounding the shoulders by pinching your shoulder blades together.

Variations:

- Assume a seated position, but don't round your low back.
- Perform this exercise while lying face down.

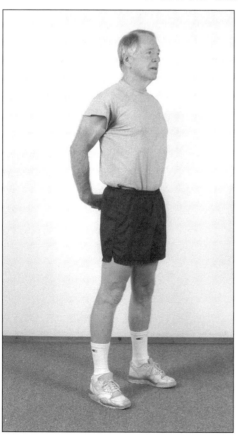

- In either a seated, standing, or prone (lying face down) position, grasp a towel in each hand and lift your arms backward and up.

- From a standing position, turn your body slightly to your right and place your right hand behind you in contact with a wall or rest it on an object that supports the hand at about shoulder height. Keeping the hand supported or maintaining contact with the wall, slowly turn your upper body left, or away from your right hand. Repeat on the opposite side.

Health/Performance Purpose:
This stretch can help improve flexibility and relieve tightness in the shoulder and chest regions that results from poor daily posture and repetitive sport movements. Sitting at your desk, driving, continually reaching forward, tennis, golf, swimming, walking, and running are examples of activity that can lead to rounded shoulders and hunched-over posture. Opening up the chest by squeezing the shoulder blades together and pulling the arms back can prevent or reduce pain in the neck and improve sport performance that is limited by restricted shoulder movement and poor head alignment. Rounded shoulders and a caved-in chest can cause your neck to jut out, which can lead to chronic misalignment and pain.

stretch

2

Overhead Triceps/Shoulder Stretch

Body Parts Targeted:
Back of the shoulders and upper arms; sides of the upper body

Muscles Stretched:
Posterior deltoid and triceps; latissimus dorsi

Execution of Stretch:
Stand with your feet shoulder-width apart and knees slightly bent. Lift one arm overhead. Bend this elbow, reaching down with the hand toward the opposite shoulder blade. Walk your fingertips down your back as far as you can. Hold this position. Reach up with the opposite arm and grasp your flexed elbow. Gently assist the stretch by pulling on the elbow.

Technique and Stretch Tips:
Pull your shoulder blades slightly toward one another during the stretch and keep your elbow pointed toward the ceiling.

Variation:

- If you're unable to stretch comfortably as described, use a towel to assist you so that you can link your hands. Place the towel in the hand that is reaching overhead, as described. Rather than reach up and in front of your body with your other hand, take that hand and reach behind your back until you can grasp the towel that is dangling down from the upper hand. Pull gently on the towel to assist the stretch.

Health/Performance Purpose:
This stretch can help improve flexibility and relieve tightness in the shoulder and back regions that results from poor daily posture and repetitive sport movements.

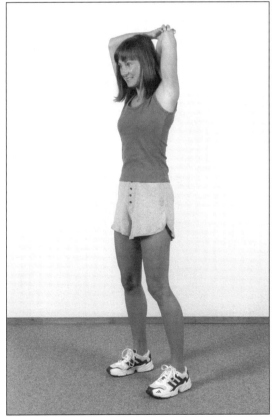

stretch 3

Arm-Across Shoulder Stretch

Body Parts Targeted:
Back of the shoulders and upper arms; upper back and sides of the body

Muscles Stretched:
Posterior deltoid and triceps; latissimus dorsi

Execution of Stretch:
Stand with your feet a comfortable distance apart, your knees slightly bent, and your toes pointing forward. Raise the left arm in front of you to shoulder height. Reach across your body with this arm and with your right hand, coming from below the raised left arm, grasp just above the left elbow with the opposite hand. As you assist the left arm across the body with your right hand, keep the arm you're stretching parallel to the ground. Repeat on the other side.

Technique and Stretch Tips:
Pull the arm slowly across the body until you feel a gentle stretch in the back of the shoulder, upper arm, and upper back muscles. Do not rotate your upper body or knees. Instead, keep your shoulders, hips, and knees facing forward as you pull the arm across. Do not round your low back during the stretch.

Variations:
- Assume the same starting position and move the arm being stretched forward and up.
- Assume the same starting position and reach forward with both arms, just below

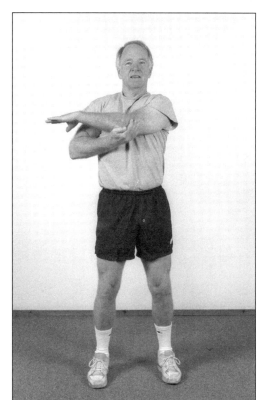

shoulder height. Grasp your left wrist with your right hand. Without rotating your body, pull your left arm out and across toward the right side of your body. You'll feel the stretch through the back of your shoulder and upper arm, as well as along the entire left side of the upper body and middle of your back. Repeat on the other side.

Health/Performance Purpose:
This stretch can help improve flexibility and relieve tightness in the shoulder, neck, and back regions that result from poor daily posture and repetitive sport movements.

stretch
4

Arm Press-Down Stretch

Body Parts Targeted:

Back of the shoulders and upper arms; sides of the body

Muscles Stretched:

Posterior deltoid and triceps; latissimus dorsi

Execution of Stretch:

Locate a stable house fixture or piece of equipment that is about hip height (examples include stationary bikes, other exercise equipment, and secure stair banisters). Move your feet about an arm's length from the fixture and stand with your feet at hip width or slightly wider. Your knees are slightly bent and your toes are pointing forward or can be slightly turned out. Reach forward and place both hands on the fixture. Move your hips back and allow your elbows to straighten as you settle into the stretch.

Technique and Stretch Tips:

Relax into this stretch by allowing your arms to straighten. You won't get the feeling of a weightless hang unless you allow your weight to move back and your arms need to straighten. Think about pressing your underarms into the ground and do not round your low back during the stretch. Keep a little tension in your abdominal muscles.

Variation:

• Use different height fixtures and/or place your hands higher or lower.

Health/Performance Purpose:

This stretch can help improve flexibility and relieve tightness in the shoulder and back regions that result from poor daily posture and repetitive sport movements.

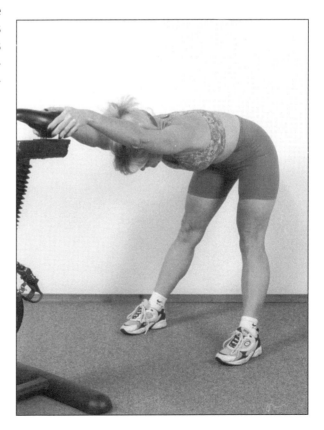

stretch
5

Arm Press-Down/Inner Thigh Stretch

Body Parts Targeted:

Back of the shoulder and upper arm; sides of the body; inner thighs

Muscles Stretched:

Posterior deltoid and triceps; latissimus dorsi; adductor (inner thigh) muscles

Execution of Stretch:

(The first part of this stretch is the same as stretch #4.)

Locate a stable house fixture or piece of equipment that is about hip height (examples include stationary bikes, other exercise equipment, and secure stair banisters). Move your feet about an arm's length from the fixture and stand with your feet at hip width or slightly wider. Your knees are slightly bent and your toes are pointing forward or can be slightly turned out. Reach forward and place both hands on the fixture. Move your hips back and allow your elbows to straighten as you settle into the stretch. To stretch the inner thighs, slowly shift your hips from this starting, centered position toward and over your right foot. The right knee may bend slightly and you'll feel the stretch in your left inner thigh (keep this leg straight). Move back through center position, pause for a moment, and then move your hips over the other foot.

Technique and Stretch Tips:

Relax into this stretch by allowing your arms to straighten. You won't get the feeling of a weightless hang unless you allow your weight to move back and your arms to straighten. Think about pressing your underarms into the ground and do not round your low back during the stretch. As you move side to side to stretch the inner thighs, keep the movement controlled and minimize any bending of the knees.

Variation:

• Keep it simple on this one. The best height for stretching the inner thighs is about hip height, so no variety for the sake of variety!

Health/Performance Purpose:

This dynamic stretch can help improve flexibility and relieve tightness in the shoulder and back regions that results from poor daily posture and repetitive sport movements. This stretch also allows you to stretch the inner thighs without doing a higher-risk, side-to-side, deep-lunge movement.

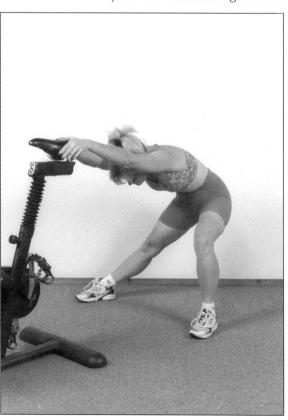

Outer Hip Push-Away Stretch

Body Parts Targeted:
Sides of the hips (outer hip)

Muscles Stretched:
Gluteus medius and minimus (hip abductor muscles); tensor fascia latae

Execution of Stretch:
Locate a stable house fixture or piece of equipment that is about hip height. Stand next to the fixture with your feet at hip width or narrower. Your knees are straight, but not locked, and your toes are pointing forward. Reach to the side with your inside hand (closest to the fixture) and grasp the fixture. Take your outside hand and place it on the fixture to the outside of the other hand. Now, bend your inside knee slightly and push your opposite hip directly out to the side, away from the fixture. The weight of your body is on the outside leg. Repeat stretch on the other side.

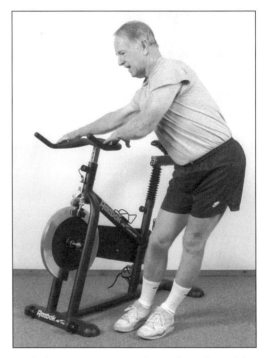

Technique and Stretch Tips:
Keep your feet close to the fixture and about hip-width apart. Form a C-curve with the side of the body that is closest to the fixture. Keep the knee of the hip being stretched fairly straight and the weight of the body on this leg.

Variations:
- To intensify the stretch, open (turn) the hip that is being stretched away from the center of your body.
- To intensify the stretch, take your inside leg and cross it in front of the leg being stretched. Bear most of your weight on the hip being stretched. Contact the tip of the toe of the non-weight-bearing leg (the one you crossed in front) on the floor for balance.
- Combine the first two variations.
- This stretch can easily be performed without a stabilizing fixture. Simply stand with your feet close together, bend one knee slightly, and shift your hips to one side, extending one hip out past the ankle until you feel a gentle stretch in the outer hip. Repeat on the other side.

Health/Performance Purpose:
This stretch can improve flexibility and relieve tightness in the sides of the hip and outer thigh regions that result from poor daily posture and repetitive sport movements that require limited range of motion (such as walking, running, and cycling). This stretch can also help reduce the likelihood of an overuse injury. Don't use this stretch if you've had hip replacement surgery or have bad hips until you've gotten your doctor's OK.

Quad/Hip Flexor Stretch

Body Parts Targeted:

Front of the thigh and hip

Muscles Stretched:

Quadriceps and hip flexors (rectus femoris, iliacus, psoas)

Execution of Stretch:

Stand close to a bench, chair, wall, or other solid object. Assist your balance with one hand. Bend one knee and lift your heel toward the buttocks. Reach back with your same side hand and grasp the top of your foot. Keeping the inner thighs close together, slowly pull your heel toward your buttocks until you feel a gentle stretch in the front of your thigh (quadriceps muscle). To stretch your hip flexors, draw your leg back (extend the hip) by tightening the buttocks muscle. Then, tighten your abdominals and attempt to roll your hips under you. This technique creates more stretch in the front of the hip (hip flexors). Repeat with your other leg.

Technique and Stretch Tips:

Contract your abdominal muscles to avoid arching your low back during the first part of this stretch. Keep your kneecap pointing straight down and oriented to the floor during the stretch. Be sure that your knees are close together. If you allow the knee of the leg being stretched to move outward, this puts stress on the medial (inside) ligaments of the knee. Always use the same side hand to pull the heel toward the buttocks. This avoids lateral (side-to-side) stress to the knee. The knee is a hinge joint and can be injured more easily when lateral forces are applied. An effective quad and hip flexor stretch does not mean that the heel must come in contact with your buttocks. The goal is to stretch muscle tissue, not touch your buttocks with your heel.

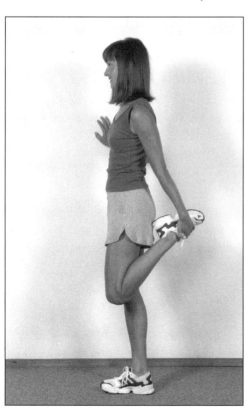

Variations:

• Try this stretch lying on your side or face down. Technique does not change.

• Emphasize grasping the top of the foot and pulling the bottom of the foot toward the buttocks. This will give you a good stretch in the front of the lower leg (shin).

Health/Performance Purpose:

This stretch can improve flexibility and relieve tightness in the front of the thigh and hip that results from poor daily posture and repetitive sport movements that require limited range of motion (such as walking, running, and cycling).

Standing Hip Flexor Stretch

Body Parts Targeted:

Front of the thigh and hip

Muscles Stretched:

Hip flexors and, to some degree, the quadriceps

Execution of Stretch:

Stand to the side of a chair, wall, or other solid object and assist your balance with one hand. Position your feet so that one foot is in front of the other, or astride. The feet should be placed hip-width apart. Keep your head, shoulders, and hips aligned over one another, and keep your chest lifted by slightly pulling your shoulder blades together. Move your hips forward and bend your front leg without changing your foot position. Roll your hips under you without flattening your low back by lightly tightening your abdominals until you feel mild tension in the front of your back leg. Repeat with your other leg.

Technique and Stretch Tips:

Maintain an upright posture. Do not bend over from the waist and keep your back leg straight. Once you've assumed your astride stance, one foot in front of the other, keep your feet about hip-width apart. This will help your balance. Bend your front knee as you move your hips forward into the stretch. Avoid arching your back by keeping your abdominal muscles contracted. Tightening your abs will also help stretch the hip.

Variation:

- Stand upright and perform the stretch without balance assistance.

Health/Performance Purpose:

This stretch can improve flexibility and relieve tightness in the front of the thigh and hip that results from poor daily posture and repetitive sport movements. The hip flexors also tend to be very tight because of prolonged and frequent sitting, which reflects a workplace reality for many people. Tight hip flexors can cause the pelvis to shift forward, creating a chronic arch (swayback) in the low back. This can lead to low back pain and discomfort.

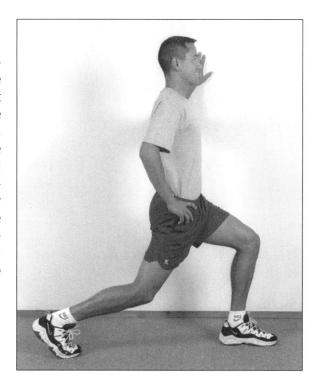

stretch 9

Standing Hamstrings Stretch

Body Part Targeted:

Back of the thigh

Muscle Stretched:

Hamstrings

Execution of Stretch:

Stand on a level surface. Extend one leg out in front of you. Keep the bottom of the foot in contact with the ground. With your hands resting lightly on the front of your thighs, bend your back knee and lean forward slightly until you feel a stretch in the back of the thigh (hamstrings muscle). Be sure to hinge from your hip joint rather than bending (rounding) at your waist or spine. As you lean forward with the upper body, feel as if you are sitting back into an invisible chair. Repeat with your other leg.

Technique and Stretch Tips:

When you lean from your hip, place your hands above the knee that is extended in front of you or place it on the other thigh. This will prevent you from putting unnecessary pressure on the knee. Do not round at the waist as you lean forward. Hinge from the hip. Once you've assumed your astride stance, one foot in front of the other, keep your feet about hip-width apart. This will help your balance.

Variations:

- Perform the stretch with your front leg placed on an elevated surface. For example, use a table, step, park bench, or chair that is not higher than a foot or two. Point the toe of this elevated leg.

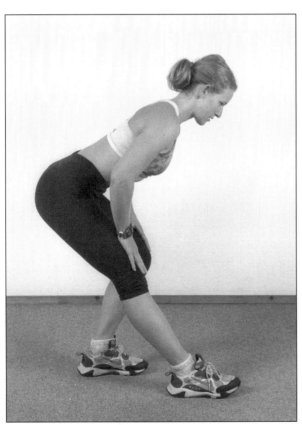

- To stretch the calf, perform the stretch as described, but instead of keeping the foot in front flat (pointed), pull the toe toward you by using the muscles in the front of your shin. Then, lean slowly forward with the torso. You'll feel the difference. Be sure to stretch the other calf, too.

Health/Performance Purpose:

This stretch can help improve flexibility and relieve tightness in the back of the thigh that results from poor daily posture and repetitive sport movements. This muscle can become tight if you sit a lot, especially with a rounded low back. Not only is this poor posture stressful to your spinal discs and ligaments, it can also lead to a chronically flexed or rounded low back posture. This flat-back posture, combined with tight hip flexors, can lead to limited pelvic movement. This in turn can result in low back pain and discomfort. (And, if your hips are frozen, you can't dance!)

Standing Gluteal Stretch

Body Parts Targeted:

Buttocks and outer hip

Muscles Stretched:

Gluteus maximus (primarily)

Execution of Stretch:

Locate a stable house fixture or piece of equipment that is about hip height (stationary bikes, other equipment, and secure stair banisters). Move your feet about an arm's length from the fixture and stand with your feet at hip width or slightly wider. Reach forward and place both hands on the fixture.

Now, move one foot slightly forward and toward the center of your body, toes pointing forward. Lift the other leg off the ground by bending your knee and rotating

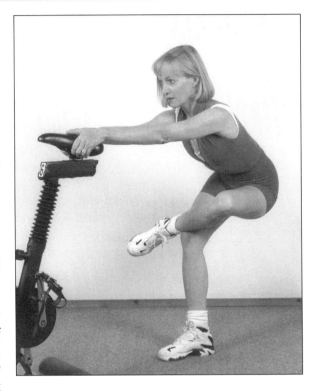

your thigh outward. Place the ankle of the rotated and lifted leg just above the knee of the support leg (this forms the number 4). Move your hips back and bend the knee of the leg you're standing on. Allow your elbows to straighten as you settle into the stretch. Repeat on the other leg.

Technique and Stretch Tips

You won't get the feeling of a weightless hang unless you allow your weight to move back and your arms to straighten. Think about pressing your underarms into the ground and do not round your low back during the stretch. Bend the knee of the support leg only as deeply as is comfortable.

Variations:

- Increase the stretch by rotating your thigh open more, without assistance.
- Increase the stretch by rotating your thigh open more with the assistance of your same-side hand.
- Increase the stretch by bending the knee of the support leg deeper. (The thigh should go no deeper than parallel to the floor.)

Health/Performance Purpose:

This stretch can improve flexibility and relieve tightness in the outer hip and buttocks regions that results from poor daily posture and repetitive sport movements like those in running, cycling, and walking. These muscles can become tight if you don't stretch them regularly, which can lead to overuse injuries.

stretch 11

Standing Calf Stretch

Body Part Targeted:

Back of the lower leg (calves)

Muscles Stretched:

Gastrocnemius and soleus

Execution of Stretch:

Stand approximately one arm's length away from a wall, chair, or tree. Move one foot in close to the chair while extending the other leg behind you. Keep your feet about hip-width apart. With the leg closest to the chair bent and your back leg straight, place your hands on the chair. Keep the back heel on the ground with the knee straight and move your hips forward. The toes of both feet remain pointed forward. Slowly lean forward from the ankle, keeping your back straight until you feel a stretch in the calf muscles. Repeat with your other leg.

Technique and Stretch Tips:

Lean forward from your ankles and not your waist as you shift your hips forward. This is called a straight-body lean. The ears, shoulders, hips, and support leg ankle are aligned. Keep the back heel on the ground and the back leg straight. Keep your feet shoulder-width apart. This will assist your balance.

Variations:

- Try the same stretch without balance assistance. Stand upright, step forward, and place your hands on the thigh of your front leg.
- Perform the stretch described, but bend the back leg to target the stretch in the soleus muscle.
- See stretch #9, second variation.

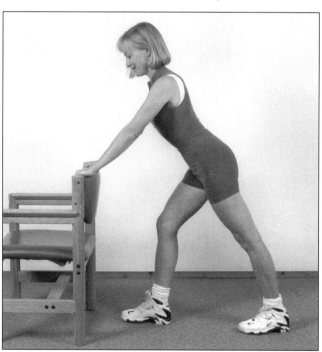

Health/Performance Purpose:

This stretch can improve flexibility and relieve tightness in the lower leg. The calves can become tight as a result of wearing high heels, walking, running, cycling, and maintaining standing posture for long periods of time. These postural muscles become tight if you don't stretch them regularly, which can lead to overuse injuries.

stretch

12

Shin Stretch

Body Part Targeted:

Front of the lower leg (anterior compartment muscles)

Muscle Stretched:

Tibialis anterior (primarily)

Execution of Stretch:

Stand to the side of a chair or wall and assist your balance with one hand. One foot is in front of the other. Keep your head, shoulders, and hips aligned and keep your chest lifted by slightly pulling your shoulder blades together. Now, place all of your weight on the forward leg. Point the toe of your back leg and point your shoelaces toward the ground. Gently press the top of the foot and ankle into the ground as your front leg bends. Move your hips forward without changing your foot position until you feel mild tension in the front of your shin. Repeat with the other leg.

Technique and Stretch Tips:

Do not bend over from the waist. Once you've assumed your astride stance, keep your feet about hip-width apart. Avoid arching your back by keeping your abdominal muscles contracted. Imagine you are pressing the back leg ankle and top of the foot into the ground and simultaneously pulling it forward. (The back foot does not actually travel forward, but envision this to help you effectively stretch.)

Variation:

- Crossovers. Stand upright and cross the right foot over the left foot. Place the right foot so it's just outside the left ankle and the shoelaces of the right shoe are facing toward the ground (the bottom of the right foot should not be in contact with the ground). Gently press the left knee into the calf until mild tension is felt in the right shin area. Hold and repeat on the other side.

Health/Performance Purpose:

To improve flexibility and relieve tightness in the front of the lower leg that results from repetitive movements. These muscles are required to lift the toe, especially during walking, so that the foot clears the ground and you don't stumble. The muscles of the shin can become tight if you don't stretch them regularly and can contribute to overuse injuries (for example, shin splints) and poor performance.

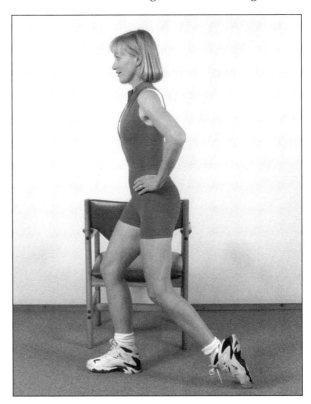

Back Curl Stretch

Body Part Targeted:

Low back (lumbar region)

Muscles Stretched:

Erector spinae and quadratus lumborum

Execution of Stretch:

Kneel on all fours with your hands directly below your shoulders and knees below your hips. Keep your neck straight. Gently pull your shoulder blades toward one another. Your low back is neither flat nor extremely arched. Tighten your abdominals and roll your hips under you. Hold this rounded low back position for a moment and return to your starting, or neutral, position.

Technique and Stretch Tips:

Don't round your upper back. Keep your shoulder blades pulled together during the entire stretch. The only movement occurs between your ribs and the top of your hips.

Variations:

- Lie on your back with your head and feet on the ground and your knees bent. Pull one knee toward the chest, hold the stretch, and lower your leg. Repeat with the other leg.

- Lie flat on your back with your head and feet in contact with the ground and your knees bent. Pull both knees toward the chest. Pause and hold the stretch. Lower one leg, then the other. (Lowering both legs simultaneously can strain the low back.)

Health/Performance Purpose:

This stretch can improve flexibility and relieve tightness in the low back that can result from continual contraction of these postural muscles. If your back is excessively arched, strong abdominals can control the degree of arch. This stretch exercise may best serve as an abdominal strengthener.

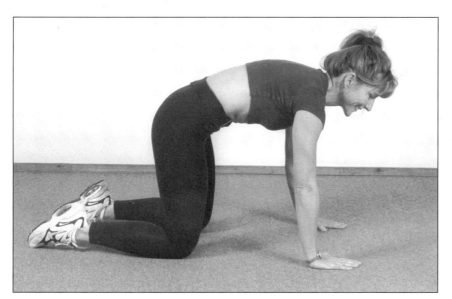

Rarely, in today's society of an automated workplace and hours spent at a desk job or computer, is the low back area tight. Instead, these muscles are usually over-stretched! Maintain a slight, natural curve in your low back when you sit, stand, and move. Don't let your low back round for extended periods of time.

stretch

14

Back Arch (or Extension) Stretch

Body Parts Targeted:

Abdominals (front of trunk between the ribs and top of the hip)

Muscles Stretched:

Abdominals (rectus abdominis and obliques)

Execution of Stretch:

Kneel on all fours with your hands directly below your shoulders and knees positioned below your hips. Keep your neck straight (neither lifted or dropped). Gently pull your shoulder blades toward one another. Your low back is neither flat nor extremely arched (neutral position). Tighten your low back muscles and arch your low back (push your belly button toward the floor). Hold this arched low back position and return to your starting, or neutral, position.

Technique and Stretch Tips:

Don't round your upper back. Keep your shoulder blades pulled together during the entire stretch. The only movement occurs between your ribs and the top of your hips.

Variation:

• Combine this stretch with stretch #13. This combination creates an excellent pelvic mobility exercise, as well as an ab and back strengthener.

Health/Performance Purpose:

Probably more important than stretching your abdominals (though it feels good and maintains range of motion), this stretch can be an important first step in strengthening the low back muscles. As mentioned in stretch #13, more often than not, the low back muscles need to be strengthened, rather than stretched. Low back pain or discomfort can result from weak and overstretched spinal muscles, so this exercise is a good way to increase low back muscle endurance. To avoid hurting your spine, maintain a slight, natural curve in your low back when you sit, stand, and move. Don't let your low back fall into an excessively arched position simply because of poor posture awareness.

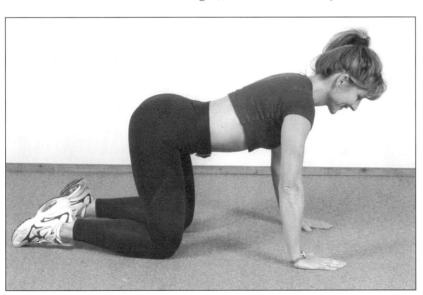

Lateral Head Tilt Stretch

Body Parts Targeted:
Sides and back of neck

Muscles Stretched:
Neck extensors and lateral flexors

Execution of Stretch:
Stand with your feet hip-width apart and knees slightly bent. Let your arms hang relaxed by your sides. Slowly move your right ear toward your right or same-side shoulder. Simultaneously press your left hand toward the floor and your left shoulder away from your left ear. Do this slowly and with control until you feel mild tension in the left side of your neck, shoulder, and upper back. Hold this position, then release the arm that is pressing down, return your head to its starting position, and then repeat the stretch on the other side.

Technique and Stretch Tips:
Tilt your head directly to the side, not forward or back. Use control when pressing your shoulder down to intensify the stretch. If you're already getting a nice stretch after you tilt the neck, omit the shoulder and hand press.

Variations:
- Perform the stretch, but vary your head position slightly forward, rather than tilting it directly to the side.
- Head rotations. Rotate your head side to side by looking over one shoulder, then the other. Keep your chin level or parallel to the floor and your hip and shoulders facing forward.

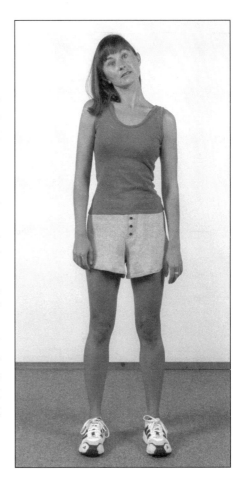

Health/Performance Purpose:
This stretch can improve flexibility and relieve tightness and tension in the sides and back of the neck. Tension in this area of the body results from poor daily posture while, for example, seated at a desk or driving, and during repetitive sport movements (such as swimming, biking, or in-line skating). If your head is positioned properly, your neck should be absent of tension, meaning it is neither forward, back, nor tilted to the side. Take stretch breaks regularly when you're on the job or working out and check your neck posture regularly. (Use a mirror to help you get a feel for this neutral, tension-free position.)

5 Strengthen Your Heart

Although exercise to challenge the cardiovascular system may seem like the simple part of your exercise program, that's not necessarily the case. Understanding why you participate in the cardio activities you do can help you avoid boredom while simultaneously improving your results and giving your mind a break. And, knowing how to change your program and what level of effort to work out at will maximize your cardiovascular training time.

You'll realize, too, that you have three different energy systems (one aerobic and two anaerobic) that work together to fuel optimal cardiovascular performance. Both the aerobic and anaerobic systems need to be trained. The aerobic system generally manufactures energy for low- to moderate-level intensity exercise. If you're highly trained it can even sustain high-intensity activity. Consider a competitive runner who keeps a five-minute pace per mile for 26 miles! Aerobic effort is relative to your personal cardiovascular fitness level. A five-minute-mile pace that would drop most runners into an exhausted pile of heaving breaths is a very manageable submaximal effort for highly conditioned endurance athletes.

The aerobic system helps you recover from fatigue that results from fairly hard to all-out and short-duration anaerobic exercise. A strong aerobic base lays a training foundation that allows you to work longer at higher, yet manageable, intensities and still remain predominantly aerobic. At higher levels of effort you'll be able to postpone fatigue and recover more quickly.

The two anaerobic systems produce energy to meet activity demands that call for intense, immediate, and relatively short-duration periods. The aerobic system is not capable of providing energy for intense activity that is of short duration. Ten repetitions performed to fatigue, a 100-meter sprint performed all-out, a quick pivot or leap, or a 30-second burst of speed during a run represent examples of activities that use anaerobic energy contributions during exercise.

KEY POINT

It's important to prepare both the aerobic and anaerobic energy systems to meet the demands of your training and daily life. Ultimately, all activity depends on the aerobic energy system to produce energy and replenish exhausted energy stockpiles.

Most types of cells—including those of the heart, nerves, and brain—can produce energy only aerobically. That is why a constant supply of oxygen to these cells is necessary. For example, if the delivery of oxygen to a portion of the heart is stopped, that area of the heart suffers a heart attack or myocardial infarction. If the brain stops getting oxygen, a stroke occurs in the deprived area. Nearly all cells in the body require a constant supply of oxygen.

On the other hand, the muscles of your body can create energy with (aerobic) or without (anaerobic) oxygen. However, the muscles recover from anaerobic work such as strength training or a hard sprint, only when enough oxygen (aerobic energy production) is available during recovery after the hard effort. Oxygen must be available so that the depleted anaerobic energy stores such as adenosine triphosphate (ATP) and creatine phosphate (CP), can be replenished. So you see, even anaerobic exercise is ultimately dependent on the ability of your body to deliver and use oxygen.

When you say you're "aerobic" or "anaerobic," these words actually refer to the *muscles being used for the activity.* This is true since the energy for muscle contraction and movement is produced *inside* the muscle cells. In reality, your body is *always* aerobic, until your last gasp! From this perspective you probably prefer to remain aerobic for a long time! And yes, you're aerobic at rest. However, because your energy output is so low, this is not a very effective way to burn calories and fat and get into shape.

Aerobic exercise is the key to building a stronger heart that can reduce your chances of heart disease, burn lots of fat, and deliver oxygen to the cells of your body for continuous activity or recovery from hard effort. Aerobic exercise is any activity that you can keep at for about two minutes or longer that raises your heart rate and generally involves the large muscle groups of the hips, thighs, and buttocks.

Aerobic exercise means that your muscles are getting enough oxygen to make energy by aerobic energy production. When you produce energy aerobically, generally you can carry on a conversation while exercising and you feel like you could continue exercising indefinitely. (On the other hand, if you can recite the Gettysburg address with theatrics and gusto, maybe you should work a little harder!)

Anaerobic exercise occurs when the exercising muscles no longer get enough oxygen to produce the necessary energy aerobically and you must rely on the anaerobic system. The more fit you are, the more capable your cardiovascular system is of delivering adequate oxygen to keep up aerobic energy production at harder levels of intensity. This means you can work harder and burn more calories at high levels of effort that are still tolerable to you. At some point, however, things get tough. You start to breathe harder and more rapidly, you can't speak a short sentence without gasping, and your muscles start to burn. You are approaching your anaerobic threshold (lactate threshold), which is the point at which lactic acid production and accumulation is greater than its removal. At some point, lactic acid buildup in the muscle temporarily interferes with working muscles and leads to fatigue. During recovery, the aerobic system delivers oxygen, and the lactic acid is used for energy and removed.

Is anaerobic exercise bad? Remember, the anaerobic systems allow you to work above a submaximal or steady pace. But the temporary accumulation of lactic acid is the price you pay for the ability to sustain more intense effort. A better question might be, Is anaerobic energy system training appropriate to my goals and can I modify this type of exercise to meet my needs? You'll find that the answer to both of these questions is yes.

KEY POINT

A healthy cardiovascular system that is challenged by aerobic activity and not compromised by a poor diet ensures an adequate supply and use of oxygen for most of the body's functions. Aerobic conditioning moves your body toward being a more efficient machine in relation to its ability to carry out everyday tasks, recreation, and sport and still have energy to burn when your day ends.

BENEFITS OF AEROBIC TRAINING

Aerobic exercise that increases your heart rate and lasts longer than a few minutes gives you a performance edge, burns lots of calories, and confers many health benefits. Not only is it important to keep the cardiovascular system in top shape from a performance perspective, but health implications with regard to aerobic training loom importantly, too.

Health benefits of aerobic exercise include the following:

1. A stronger and healthier heart.
2. Increased HDL. This "good" cholesterol helps keep your arteries unplugged and healthy.
3. Decreased total cholesterol. This is the debris in your blood that can clog your arteries.
4. Reduced blood pressure. Even moderate exercise can help.
5. Reduced risk for heart attack and stroke.
6. Decreased body fat and an ability to help maintain your desirable weight. You'll become a better fat-burner and burn a lot of calories every session.
7. Decreased risk for diabetes.
8. Reduced feelings of anxiety, tension, and depression. When these feelings creep into your life, reach for the exercise cure.

9. Improved sleep. When you train hard, you need quality rest.

10. Higher levels of energy. Efficient delivery and use of blood and oxygen is the key to increased vigor and performance.

HOW THE AEROBIC SYSTEM WORKS

The cardiovascular system is a transport network in the body. *Cardio* refers to the heart and its pumping force that circulates the blood through an amazing network of blood vessels. *Respiratory* refers to the lungs and the exchange of gases. Oxygen and carbon dioxide are two important gases exchanged in the lungs, as well as in the cells of the body.

The cardiovascular system consists of the heart, lungs, arteries (carrying oxygen-loaded blood away from the heart throughout the body), capillaries (exchanging gases, nutrients, and by-products between the bloodstream and cells), and veins (carrying oxygen-depleted blood back to the heart). An important purpose of the cardiovascular system is to deliver oxygen to the various tissues of the body, both at rest and during a broad spectrum of exercise intensities, from low level to high level.

Blood is the vehicle that delivers oxygen and nutrients (such as fat and carbohydrates) to the cells in the body where they are needed to produce ATP (the energy necessary for muscle contraction). Blood also picks up metabolic by-products (the leftovers) of energy metabolism, including lactic acid, water, and carbon dioxide. In contrast to a waste product that has no usefulness and is difficult to dispose of, by-products such as carbon dioxide can be carried easily to the lungs and exhaled out of the body, and water can be sweated out of the body or exhaled (expelled air is loaded with humidity or water). In addition, blood carries lactic acid to the liver where it is metabolized (oxidized) when enough oxygen is available and used for energy.

Lactic acid is *not* a waste product. Its production at higher intensity levels (such as when performing interval training or exercising beyond your "cruise" or comfort zone) allows you to work out at harder levels than can be sustained with aerobic metabolism. During recovery, or when the activity is slowed, sufficient oxygen becomes available again and lactic acid is oxidized (broken down) and eventually used as an energy source.

> ## KEY POINT
> Scientific fact and understanding should dictate training protocol. With accurate knowledge you can plan and confidently follow your training program.

Energy for Cardiovascular Conditioning

Think of your body as a factory. It processes different raw materials to make its final product, which is energy (ATP). Energy is used by every cell in the body, including your muscles (muscle cells). Oxygen, carbohydrates (sugar and starches), fat, and protein are the raw materials available to your body in virtually an unlimited supply to create ATP, or energy for movement.

ATP is used as the energy supply for muscles and other body functions. When a muscle contracts and exerts force, the energy used to drive the contraction comes from ATP. However, since the amount of ATP stored in the muscle is small, your body begins to produce more ATP immediately by breaking down carbohydrate and fat in the presence of oxygen. (Sustained aerobic activity, such as a 35-minute run or cycle, is a good example of this type of energy production.) The duration of activity would be severely limited if the body was not able to produce ATP aerobically, or as it is needed for low-level to vigorous exercise. ATP is ultimately the body's only energy source and is supplied both aerobically and anaerobically, depending on the intensity of the activity.

To understand how a muscle cell produces energy for cardiovascular effort, it's important to view the three primary energy systems of the body (two anaerobic and one aerobic) as complements of one another. These three systems are used more or less, depending on what kind of energy production is required by a particular aerobic or anaerobic activity.

Aerobic means "with oxygen." Energy is produced aerobically as long as *enough* oxygen is supplied to the exercising muscles by the cardiovascular system. Even when the cardiovascular system is unable to supply enough oxygen, your muscles can still produce energy via a process called anaerobic metabolism. The muscles produce energy without oxygen, or more accurately, without sufficient oxygen.

The anaerobic system produces energy via two systems. The immediate energy system is called the adenosine triphosphate/creatine phosphate (ATP-CP) system. This stored energy in the body's muscles is used for all-out muscular effort that lasts for about 10 seconds. ATP and CP are broken apart to release energy for these powerful efforts, but must be rejoined through aerobic energy production. The second anaerobic system, the short-term energy or lactic acid system, produces energy anaerobically at the expense of lactic acid buildup. This will eventually limit the body's ability to continue exercising (producing energy) at this higher intensity of effort. Both the ATP-CP and short-term energy (lactic acid) systems represent the two anaerobic energy systems available to your body that can contribute to anaerobic metabolism.

In intense exercise of short duration (100-yard dash, traditional resistance training where you tire after about 6 to 20 repetitions, or a quick walk up a hill), the energy is predominantly derived from the already-present stores of intra-muscular (already stored in the muscle) ATP and CP using the immediate and short-term anaerobic energy systems mentioned earlier. After several minutes, oxygen consumption becomes an important factor if the activity is to be sustained, and the predominant energy pathway is the long-term, aerobic energy system.

To develop the cardiovascular system totally, *both* aerobic and anaerobic energy systems must be trained. Regardless of whether the goal of your program is performance or reducing body fat, include both. Why? The anaerobic systems use stored ATP-CP (CP is stored to a limited extent, just like ATP, and is used to reform ATP) and burn glucose, a simple sugar derived from carbohydrates. Training the anaerobic system will allow you to work harder for longer periods of time. The aerobic system also uses glucose, but in the process it burns fat as well. Stored body fat is released into the bloodstream and sent to the muscles where, in the presence of oxygen and glucose, it is burned aerobically to produce energy. Fat can only be burned aerobically (in the presence of oxygen), and the by-products of the aerobic system—carbon dioxide and water—do not lead to quick muscle fatigue. On the other hand, burning glucose anaerobically allows you to work at a level of intensity for a short time period that you could not sustain aerobically, but it leads to the formation of lactic acid and quick fatigue. Training aerobically will also make you an efficient fat-burner.

> ### KEY POINT
>
> Aerobic or anaerobic exercise is neither good nor bad. Which type of cardiovascular exercise is appropriate to your needs and exercise goals? The answer: Both!

The more fit you are—that means training both the anaerobic and aerobic energy systems—the more capable your cardiovascular system is of delivering and using adequate oxygen to sustain aerobic energy production at increasingly higher levels of intensity. This training adaptation results in your being able to comfortably tolerate higher levels of effort for a given time period. This maximizes training benefit and calories expended.

Moving Along the Energy Spectrum

At rest your muscles are aerobic. Remember, your body is always aerobic, as the cells of the heart, brain, and nerves need a constant supply of oxygen to meet their energy demands and sustain cellular life. Rest is an exercise intensity and requires a volume of oxygen ($\dot{V}O_2$) to sustain resting-energy demands of the body. Of the total calories you expend in a given day, about 70 to 75 percent are used to support resting metabolic needs!

As exercise intensity increases from rest to walking to running six-minute miles, the demand for oxygen continues to increase. It becomes more of a challenge for the cardiovascular system to get enough oxygen to the working muscles. And, unless the muscle cells are trained to do so, they may not be able to extract oxygen that is being pumped from the heart and delivered via the vessels and blood as exercise intensity increases. At somewhere between about 50 and 85 percent of maximum aerobic capacity (depending on fitness level and specific genetic factors), the delivery to, and use of, oxygen in the exercising muscles becomes inadequate. At this point, muscles shift largely to the anaerobic energy system to support continued contractions. You've experienced this shift (your anaerobic threshold) when you've pushed your aerobic pace— your muscles started to burn, your breath came in short gasps, and you knew you'd have to slow down if you wanted to continue much longer.

The intensity at which the muscles no longer get enough oxygen (they are getting some) to produce energy predominantly by aerobic metabolism is commonly referred to as the anaerobic threshold. Crossing over the anaerobic threshold is usually accompanied by a significant increase in breathing or respiration, burning muscles (accumulation of lactic acid from anaerobic energy-system contribution), and a feeling that you would like to slow down or that you could not continue this activity at the current pace indefinitely. You probably could not string together three or four words without gasping.

While one energy system will predominate over the other, both aerobic and anaerobic energy systems are *always* working, regardless of intensity or type of activity. The aerobic system produces a great deal of energy compared to the anaerobic system. It is the predominant energy system at rest, during mild to moderate or even high-intensity activity if you are highly conditioned, and during recovery from anaerobic efforts. Also, carbon dioxide and water, the primary by-products of the aerobic system, are easily eliminated by breathing and sweating.

The anaerobic system can produce energy quickly for powerful and immediate muscle contractions—without the need for "sufficient" amounts of oxygen. However, the trade-off for immediate muscular response is susceptibility to quicker fatigue.

Even the recovery from traditional anaerobic efforts (i.e., when strength training effort results in muscle fatigue in about 90 seconds or 6 to 20 controlled repetitions or during a short, near-maximal speed increase) could not be accomplished without the aerobic energy system.

I sometimes use this fact to motivate my clients who "only want to strength train" or claim they are involved in anaerobic sports. I explain that their anaerobic strength efforts, or quick sprints down the basketball court, may be enhanced by more effective and quicker recovery as a result of aerobic conditioning.

Of course, your body does not switch over to the anaerobic system all at once—or in fact totally—but *gradually shifts gears* to produce energy at a faster rate than can aerobically be supplied. This is relative to how hard you are working and how fit you are. (For example, what is easy exercise for one individual may push another over the brink.) Any activity that can be performed at an aerobic pace can also be pushed to an anaerobic level of intensity. As you become more fit, surges of increased intensity above what is comfortable might be appropriate. This is called interval or anaerobic training.

WARMING UP AND COOLING DOWN

Warming up and cooling down are essential to a balanced and safe exercise program. Too often exercisers want to jump into the meat of their programs. They may say, "I want to get to the important stuff like making my heart stronger and lifting weights," thinking this is a better use of time. These important aspects of aerobic and anaerobic training are often considered as an afterthought, or totally left out of a training program. However, once you start using them as a regular part of your program, you'll wonder why you ever treated them as though they were poison.

A proper warm-up and cool-down can

- make your workouts safer and easier to do,
- limit the risk of unnecessary stress on your heart,
- get you ready for your activity,
- improve your stamina and endurance (you won't tire as quickly),
- decrease your risk for injury,
- increase enjoyment of your workouts, and
- help you stick with your health and fitness program.

KEY POINT

After you've experienced what a good warm-up and cool-down can do for you, you'll feel like something is missing in your workouts if you leave them out.

Warming Up

A warm-up literally warms your muscles, ligaments, and tendons so they are less likely to be injured. If you're going to run, walk, lift, or jump—warm up! Warmed-up muscles move faster and produce strength better than cold muscles. A warm-up also lubricates your joints, allowing for easier and possibly less painful movement.

Easing into your workout lets your body shift blood to where you need it— your exercising muscles. A good warm-up makes workouts more enjoyable and will keep you from tiring too quickly. And, you minimize discomfort and breathlessness at the beginning of exercise if you start out slowly. This keeps you from feeling out of control and keeps your passion for exercise strong.

Warming up is important to you before *any* kind of workout (walking, jogging, tennis, strength training, and so on). Your warm-up should be aerobic in nature and only require an easy, unforced range of motion. Never push yourself beyond a point of gentle tension or strain. Keep your movements fluid, rhythmic, and controlled. Try to pick a warm-up activity that uses the same muscles you are going to call into action during your workout. Before you jog, start with a walk or slower-than-normal jogging pace. If you're going to lift weights, use exercise that will warm your entire body, such as walking on a treadmill or riding a stationary bike. In addition to an aerobic warm-up, it's also a good idea to start with lighter weights or resistance when strength training and progress to heavier weights. Lighter resistance can serve as a warm-up by itself, but to most effectively prepare your muscles for safe, effective, and injury-free strength training, use both.

Most experts believe that warm-up exercise, especially before a strenuous effort, gradually prepares you to go all out without as great a risk for incurring injury. Examples include preparing yourself to run your fastest 10K race and accelerating immediately to race pace off the starting line, the ritual warm-up throws of a softball player preparing to enter a game, and the on-deck batter's swinging of a weighted bat.

How Long Should a Warm-Up Last?

Generally, about three to five minutes is sufficient for an effective warm-up. Extend your warm-up to 10 to 15 minutes if you work out hard from the get-go, aren't in great shape, or are past the age of 50. Your body will appreciate this extra time spent preparing the muscles, ligaments, and tendons for the upcoming activity.

How Hard Should a Warm-Up Be?

You should increase exercise intensity by raising your resting heart rate (average resting heart rates vary from 40 to 75 beats per minute) to about 90 to 120 beats per minute *before* moving on to harder aerobic exercise. On the 10-point effort scale (more about this later), a warm-up should slowly increase to a level 2 to 3, which indicates a "somewhat easy" to "moderate" effort.

Sport enthusiasts at all levels often use warm-up activity to prepare themselves mentally for their event. Some evidence supports the contention that a warm-up specific to the activity itself improves the necessary skill and coordination. Sports that require accuracy, timing, and precise movements generally benefit from some type of specific warm-up or formal preliminary practice. Examples include softball, track and field, hockey, dance, gymnastics, and diving.

KEY POINT

An effective warm-up can take as little as three to five minutes at somewhat easy to moderate effort.

Cooling Down

After a good workout it is tempting to head for the nearest exit, speed through a shower, and throw yourself headlong into your work day. Don't do it! A cool-down *reverses* what your warm-up accomplished, and it's just as important to ease out of your workout as it is to ease into it. The purpose of a cool-down is to safely, and with the least amount of stress to your heart, return your body to a pre-exercise level of exertion.

If you were jogging, slow your pace to a walk and then to an easy stroll. You're at the right pace when you can easily carry on a conversation without gasping. Your cool-down should last from 5 to 10 minutes. Your heart rate should drop to about 100 beats per minute (2 to 3 on the 10-point effort scale which compares with a "somewhat easy" to "moderate" level of exertion), and you should feel like your breathing is back to normal.

The return to resting level after, say, walking to the grocery store, is hardly noticeable. But, during strenuous activity you'll notice how hard you're breathing, how much you're sweating, and that it takes a while for your breathing to slow down and the sweat to stop pouring. Here are some of the benefits of cool-down:

- Gives your heart a chance to gradually slow down
- Lets your body temperature lower (you don't want to be dripping sweat back in the office)
- Keeps blood from collecting in your legs, which could cause you to faint
- Helps in faster removal of postexercise lactic acid (you recover quicker)
- May help you avoid dizziness and that sick-to-your-stomach feeling
- In combination with stretching can reduce the likelihood of muscle soreness by preventing muscle spasms
- Provides an excellent time to add stretching exercises and acknowledge personal exercise accomplishments (i.e., short-term goals)

How Easy Should a Cool-Down Be?

An active cool-down of moderate to mild exercise means that you *continue* exercising at an intensity lower than that used during the main part of your cardiovascular conditioning workout. This easy level of effort will promote blood flow through the blood vessels and heart during recovery. With a proper active (keep moving) cool-down, your heart will work less (fewer beats per minute) and require less oxygen. This type of cool-down is more likely to prevent unnecessary physiological (i.e., breathing discomfort or heart attack if by chance you have undiagnosed heart disease) or psychological stress ("I hate working out because exercise feels so stressful").

> ### KEY POINT
>
> A cool-down should consist of gradually lessening intensity and should last at least five minutes.

Using a low-level, rhythmic activity during the cool-down allows the body to reverse the blood shunt, or shift, that occurred as you began your activity, which helps ensure adequate blood flow to the working muscles. A normal reduction of exercise intensity will be reflected by the return of exercise heart rate or perceived exertion—rather quickly—to lower levels and eventually to your pre-exercise level.

How Long Should a Cool-Down Last?

You should attain a recovery heart rate of approximately 120 beats per minute (bpm) in about three minutes (or a level of perceived exertion on the 1 to 10 effort scale of 2 to 3, which rates as a "somewhat easy" to "moderate" level of effort). After about five minutes, a heart rate of around 100 bpm should be attained. A quick recovery is dependent on your current fitness level, the intensity of effort for the preceding workout, as well as the appropriateness and intensity (make it easy if you want to recover) of the cool-down activity.

Postexercise Glow

You may know the feeling. You just finished your workout, you feel great, and your cheeks are glowing a soft red. A good cool-down gives you a psychological break to savor the great feelings of postexercise accomplishment or glow. In other words, a cool-down period is an effective time to personally acknowledge the quite significant accomplishments you have just achieved. It is also a good time to ask, How do I feel at this very instant? Most feel at least better than they did before the workout began, and many feel wonderful.

Regardless, don't cheat your body and your head (mental health and motivation) out of a cool-down. Too often, personal daily exercise accomplishments are not acknowledged because of the necessity to return to the hustle and bustle of a very scheduled life. Before you jump back into a stressful and harried routine—or even a job you love—give yourself a chance to smile and say, You know, that was a pretty good workout and I feel great! Pat yourself on the back. This time-out will go a long way with regard to keeping you motivated. Now, go ahead—dive into the shower and tackle the day head on!

TRAINING AEROBICALLY

Before the question of how long, how hard, and how often, is answered, an important concern when designing a cardiovascular program is to make sure you're applying the right overload to strengthen your heart. The right overload is defined as a rhythmic, continuous, large-muscle activity that promotes a *simultaneous* increase in heart rate and return of blood (venous return) to the heart. If continued improvements are to be realized, the overload must be progressive in nature. (That's a complex way of saying you need to work harder if you want to keep seeing progress.)

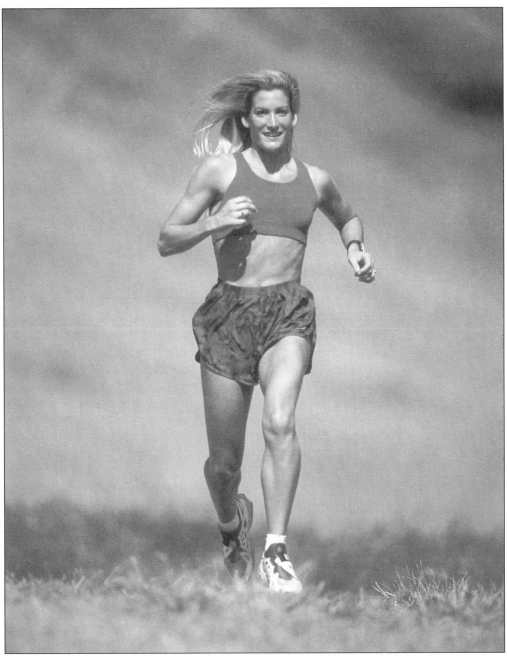

Aerobic exercise is essential for complete fitness.

Photo © Ron Dahlquist

Many factors can increase heart rate without increasing blood return to the heart. Certain drugs, excitement, stress, a hot environment, dehydration, or traditional resistance training are examples. Yet, sending a large volume of blood back to the heart is essential for a significant training effect (read this as "results") to occur in cardiovascular fitness.

Lifting moderate to heavy weights (i.e., 1 to 12 reps to fatigue) will increase your heart rate but not significantly increase your oxygen intake. This pressor response, in which heart rate increases without an equal increase in oxygen consumption and a large volume of blood does not return to the heart, occurs because the heart has to pump harder to overcome the resistance to blood flow caused by moderate to heavy exercise. If you're measuring heart rate in a situation like this, you will have a false impression that you're doing effective cardio training based on the increased heart rate. Heart rate alone will not help you answer the question, Am I doing the right kind of activity to train my cardiovascular system?

A sampling of activities that have the potential to simultaneously increase heart rate and return large volumes of blood to the heart typically involve the large muscles of the hips, thighs, and buttocks and include walking, hiking, jogging, running, cycling, in-line skating, swimming, cross-country skiing, and stair stepping.

Know Your Steady Rate

You need to know what steady-rate pace means if you want to train smart. Steady-rate exercise is a level of cardiovascular effort that is easy to maintain. You might describe this level of intensity as cruising, or characterize it by saying, I could keep this up all day long! Another good indicator of steady rate is whether or not you can sustain the pace for about two to three minutes or longer. If you fall off your exercise bike after 12 seconds, you're not working your muscles aerobically and are not at a steady rate of exercise.

It is important for you to understand how you feel during a steady-rate effort because there will be instances, such as during interval training, in which you will be encouraged to work beyond this comfort zone. Conversely, when you're recovering from vigorous exercise, you may be asked to work at or below this level. Knowing what hard or easy exercise feels like will help optimize your results. Both are equally important.

Do the Right Aerobic Activity

As mentioned, aerobic exercise is rhythmic, continuous, large-muscle (you should use the hips, thighs, and buttocks) activity. To maximize benefits and results, exercise must increase heart rate and cause a lot of blood to be pumped from, and back to, your heart. This is what conditions your heart and gives you all of those training benefits. Flexing your finger repeatedly, lifting heavy weights, or working hard pumping your channel changer (even if you use both hands) are not effective aerobic exercises because they don't cause your heart rate and the amount of blood being pumped to increase. Deep down you probably knew this to be true, but it's still a rude awakening. You know the good ones, the ones that work, and you know the right pace for aerobic activity is steady rate or below!

Besides making your heart stronger, decreasing your risk for heart disease, and burning lots of calories, how does this type of training make your body more fit? It is well documented that smart training can lead to the following changes in your body:

1. Capillary density increases with endurance-type training. This increased capillarization (which is part of your blood vessel delivery system) allows for better distribution of nutrients and oxygen to the muscles and enhanced metabolic by-product (lactic acid, carbon dioxide, water) removal.

2. The size and number of mitochondria, which are characterized as the aerobic powerhouses in the cell, increase with endurance training. This allows you to maintain a higher level of aerobic metabolism.

3. Aerobic enzymes (protein substances in the cell that facilitate energy production) increase with endurance training and enhance the ability to use oxygen more efficiently. This adaptation facilitates the energy-production process.

4. High-intensity, anaerobic interval conditioning has a positive training effect on shifting the metabolic profile of fast-twitch, Type IIa muscle fibers toward a more endurant fiber. You can train harder and longer in relative comfort (more on this in chapter 6).

5. Blood delivery (cardiac output) is improved by a stronger heart that has a greater pumping or volume capacity per heartbeat. That means that for a given effort, a trained heart can deliver the same workload with fewer heartbeats each minute.

6. Oxygen extraction (a-$\overline{v}0_2$) is improved by regular and specific training (the principle of specificity). To get better at the activity you choose, you have to participate in that activity to train the muscles involved to use the oxygen that is being delivered. Even if the heart is efficient at delivering sufficient oxygen, if the muscles are not trained to pull the oxygen from the blood stream as it travels by the muscle, performance will be limited. That's why a trained cyclist cannot elicit the same level of performance or maximal oxygen consumption if she switches to an activity she hasn't regularly trained for, such as running. With consistent and regular run training, however, the cyclist can train the muscles required of running to become better at extracting available oxygen.

Such physiological and biochemical changes in the muscle cells of the body enhance the cells' capacity to generate ATP aerobically, allowing you to work at increasingly higher levels of exercise intensity and recover more quickly from anaerobic effort. As you become more fit, as reflected by these six adaptations, these higher levels of intensity are easily accommodated by your new fitness level. You would rate the level of effort as very manageable, even though this may represent a 50 percent improvement compared to your level of fitness several months previously. This all adds up to more calories burned, maximization of time spent exercising, and enhanced performance. Plus, results will get you psyched and keep you training!

KEY POINT

Aerobic training lays the groundwork for more advanced cardiovascular training.

How Often, How Long, and How Hard

To further define cardiovascular overload (remember, you've got to choose the right kind of activity), the frequency (how often), duration (how long), and intensity (how hard) of your chosen activity must be spelled out (see table 5.1 on page 112).

How Often

If you want to see serious improvements in your fitness and develop a good training base, you need to challenge this aerobic component of fitness three to six times per week.

If you are just starting a program or are out of shape, don't let these recommendations discourage you. Instead, do your cardio training two to three times per week and wait at least a day between sessions. You'll see significant fitness improvement and health benefits. Your long-term goal is to build up to exercising on most days of the week.

How Long

How long you should work out depends on your current level of fitness. Again, if you are just starting a program, don't let the following recommendations discourage you. Instead, start with 5 to 10 minutes once or twice per day. You'll see significant fitness improvement and health benefits. Your long-term goal is to build to 30 minutes of exercise on the days you exercise.

Choose stage 1, 2, or 3 depending on your current aerobic conditioning level.

Stage 1: Conditioning Base
If you're just starting out, haven't exercised in a long time, or consider yourself out of shape, allow yourself at least four to six weeks to progress to a solid base of aerobic conditioning. You cannot progress too slowly.

Start with 5 to 15 minutes of aerobic activity such as walking or biking. The activity can be performed continuously or broken up into smaller segments such as five minutes. You could walk your dog for five minutes in the morning, take a five-minute stroll at lunch, and walk around your neighborhood in the evening. After a couple of weeks, shoot for 15 to 20 minutes per session. Remember, you can break this duration into more manageable shorter bouts of 5 to 10 minutes each and gradually work to the longer time goals.

Stage 2: Moving Beyond Base Level Fitness
If you train consistently, this stage can easily last up to six months. (Inconsistent training means you'll stay at this stage longer.) Gradually increase your duration (by about 5 to 10 percent only) every two to three weeks until you're comfortable completing 30 minutes of activity. Once again, it isn't necessary to do 30 minutes in one continuous effort to get great health and fitness results. Toward the end of this stage you can work up to an hour of total activity a couple of times per week to add variety and challenge to your workouts. Generally, exercising beyond an hour leads to diminished fitness returns (your results don't equal the effort and time you put in) and an increased risk for injury.

Stage 3: Maintenance
Maintenance of your fitness level is not regression! It's simply an acknowledgment

on your part of a personal commitment to continue your program in a fun, varied, and effective manner.

Many of you reading this book already have a high level of aerobic fitness. Reality check: once you've set the base, it's not easy to continue improving your fitness. Remember how ecstatic you were when you first started your program and your personal results cascaded in. Then, after training regularly and progressively for three to six months, those results started to trickle in. At this point, and for the rest of your life, you begin to maintain your fitness base by cross-training; adding anaerobic conditioning intervals; and varying how often, how long, and how hard you work. Remember to keep your workouts FUN! This approach will help you improve your fitness and keep you from burning out.

Maintaining your fitness level does not mean sentencing yourself to a life commitment of the same old boring routine. In fact, maintaining your fitness is far from this dreary scenario. Reaching a point of maintenance simply acknowledges your acceptance of a desired state of personal health.

KEY POINT

After any amount of sustained training (three to six months or longer), a slowdown in training benefits is inevitable. Prepare yourself in advance for this unavoidable physiological reality so that you can experience it in a positive light. The ultimate goal is to maintain your current program and level of fitness, for life!

Stage 4: Optional High-Intensity Training

You can move from maintenance periods to improving fitness by using interval training or cross-training. Regardless of which you choose, a program of periodization should always be followed (see chapters 2, 6, and 8.)

How Hard

Aerobic intensity guidelines for healthy adults are generally set at 50 to 85 percent of $\dot{V}O_2$max or heart rate reserve (HRR). $\dot{V}O_2$max is simply the maximal amount of oxygen you can breathe in every minute and is determined in a testing lab or doctor's office. Training intensities (how hard you work) are determined by taking a percentage of $\dot{V}O_2$max. A percentage of $\dot{V}O_2$max or HRR is called a target heart rate (THR). When you figure a low- and high-end percentage, this creates a target heart rate range (THRR) that you train within.

It's easier to figure out a heart rate training range (compared to obtaining a $\dot{V}O_2$max) by calculating your HRR—and this compares directly to $\dot{V}O_2$max, anyway. You can calculate HRR and your heart rate training zone in the next section, Gauging Your Efforts. If you don't like to use heart rate, use the 10-point RPE (effort) scale (Borg, G., 1982. Psychological Basis of Perceived Exertion), described in the same section, or both.

If you're deconditioned or just starting your program, don't be intimidated by these intensity recommendations. They are not written in stone. Moderate (well below the recommendations set forth) and consistent cardiovascular training can result in substantial and beneficial effects to your health and cardiovascular endurance.

Table 5.1 Progressive Cardiovascular Training Program

Conditioning Base

Week	How often (times per week)	How long (minutes)	How hard (% HRR)	How hard (RPE)	RPE descriptive rating
1	2-3	5-15	40-50	2-4	Somewhat easy to Somewhat hard
2	2-3	5-15	40-50	2-4	Somewhat easy to Somewhat hard
3	2-3	10-17	40-50	2-4	Somewhat easy to Somewhat hard
4	2-3	10-17	50-60	2-4	Somewhat easy to Somewhat hard
5	3	15-20	50-60	2-4	Somewhat easy to Somewhat hard
6	3-4	15-20	50-60	2-4	Somewhat easy to Somewhat hard

Moving Beyond Base-Level Fitness

Week	How often (times per week)	How long (minutes)	How hard (% HRR)	How hard (RPE)	RPE descriptive rating
7-9	3-4	20-25	60-65	3-4	Moderate to Somewhat hard
10-13	3-4	21-25	65-70	4-5	Somewhat hard to Hard
14-16	3-4	26-30	65-70	4-5	Somewhat hard to Hard
17-19	3-5	26-30	70-75	4-5	Somewhat hard to Hard
20-23	3-5	31-35	70-75	4-5	Somewhat hard to Hard
24-27	3-6	31-35	70-75	4-5	Somewhat hard to Hard

Maintenance

Week	How often (times per week)	How long (minutes)	How hard (% HRR)	How hard (RPE)	RPE descriptive rating
After 4-6 months	3-6	30-60	70-85	4-6	Somewhat hard to Very hard

High-Intensity Interval (optional)

Week	How often (times per week)	How long (minutes)	How hard (% HRR)	How hard (RPE)	RPE descriptive rating
After 4-6 months of steady training	1-2	See interval training (Chapter 6)	85-100	6-10	Very hard to Very very hard

Choose stage 1, 2, or 3 depending on your current aerobic conditioning base. These aerobic conditioning intensities should be complemented by anaerobic interval conditioning to reach top levels of fitness.

Stage 1: Conditioning Base

Work at a heart rate training zone between 40 and 60 percent of your heart rate reserve (HRR). This corresponds to an RPE range of 2–3 ("somewhat easy" to "moderate") to 3–4 ("moderate" to "somewhat hard"). You should be able to speak short sentences without gasping at this level of effort.

Stage 2: Moving Beyond Base Level Fitness

Work at a heart rate training zone between 60 and 75 percent of your HRR. This corresponds to an RPE range of 3 to 5 ("moderate" to "hard"). If you want higher levels of fitness, raise your training zone to 70 to 85 percent of your HRR. This corresponds to an RPE range of 4 to 6 ("somewhat hard" to "very hard"). Remember that you're doing aerobic training. Even with these increasing exercise intensities, you should still be able to pass the "talk test" by being able to speak short sentences during the activity.

Stage 3: Maintenance

Maintain your level of effort and consistency, but introduce variety. Work at both the high and low ends of the heart rate training zones and do some easy or cruiser workouts using the lower intensities in the base level stage.

Stage 4: Optional High-Intensity Training

You can move from maintenance periods to improving fitness by using interval training (85 percent and greater of your HRR) or cross-training. Regardless of which one you choose, a program of periodization should always be followed.

Smart Progression

When progressing to a higher intensity level, longer duration, or more frequent sessions, do so separately. You run the risk of overuse injury if you simultaneously increase any of these elements. A conservative, yet effective rule of thumb is not to increase any by more than about 5 percent. Adapt to this increase over a period of a week or two, and then consider changing one of the other components or progressing the one you've gotten used to, to a higher level.

The training program outlined on the previous page represents a progressive training program for cardiovascular conditioning. It can be used for any aerobic activity you choose to participate in.

GAUGING YOUR EFFORTS

The best way to monitor exercise intensity is to use a combination of heart rate monitoring and rating of perceived exertion (RPE). If you don't want to bother with heart rate monitoring, the 10-point RPE effort scale is an easy way to measure your level of effort accurately. Perceived exertion focuses on tuning into physical cues such as a quick breathing rate, breathlessness, the ability or inability to converse with short sentences during exercise or to breathe comfortably, burning muscles, and your level of fatigue during your cardiovascular training.

Finding the right level of effort is as simple as working from an easy pace to a steady-rate pace to a little harder than normal pace and, depending on your training goals, to a pace that might rate 8, 9, or 10 on a 1 to 10 effort scale. Keeping that broad range of intensities in mind, there are three simple ways to judge your intensity: the talk test, RPE (rating of perceived exertion), and heart rate measures (or counting your pulse).

Talk Test

This is the easiest way to determine how hard you're working out. To get aerobic training results and health benefits, you should work at a level of effort that is challenging, yet very sustainable. You should be able to carry on a conversation by piecing together short sentences without gasping for air, and you should be able to breathe comfortably throughout your aerobic exercise. Use the talk test as a quick check-in to see if you should slow down or speed up.

Slow down:

1. When you notice that you start breathing hard and fast. Breathing occurs in gasps and it is difficult to string together short sentences of conversation such as, I am about to die.

2. If you're close to crashing and burning. That's about to happen when your muscles start to burn and you find the exercise very uncomfortable. If you're thinking, "I can't go any longer," but can't even utter it, at least put the brakes on and slow down. You want to be challenged, but remember—you shouldn't bust your gut if aerobic training benefits are the goal.

Speed up :

1. When you can bellow out every word of your favorite songs playing through your head phones. You should be able to carry on a short conversation without being out of breath, not be able to recite the State of the Nation speech.

Rating of Perceived Exertion

Rating of perceived exertion (RPE) is an easy and practical way to monitor the levels of your aerobic (or anaerobic) workouts. RPE means you check in with how you perceive you are feeling at any given moment. Sounds weird, but it's simple. This method uses a numerical scale that ranges from 1 to 10. The numbers match with terms that describe how hard you *feel* or *think* you're working. A level 1 rating equates with vigorously manipulating your channel changer, levels 2 to 3 a cruising level of effort, and level 10 closer to vomiting.

RPE is taught by matching a number with how you feel. For example, a moderate level of effort will probably rate 2 to 3 numerically and "somewhat easy" to "moderate" descriptively. Examples of a 2 to 3 level of effort include walking or running at an easy pace and cooling down after vigorous activity. Once RPE levels are learned for each intensity level, they become a valuable tool in monitoring intensity.

The chart below will assist you in teaching yourself RPE. The numbers on this scale range from 0 to 10, with 10 representing maximal or "very, very hard" exertion.

An effective training zone corresponds to an RPE of 3 to 7 ("moderate" to "very hard"). This represents a range of intensity levels that will confer significant fitness and health benefits, as well as satisfy high-level performance goals.

Using RPE can help keep your workouts challenging and keep you getting results. Let's say you always run or walk the same course. When you first began, your RPE was 3 to 4. Now it's a 2. If you want to keep getting results, it's time to run or walk faster.

RPE is especially appropriate for you if you do not have typical heart rate response to aerobic exercise. This includes individuals who are on beta blockers (and other medications), some people with cardiac problems and diabetes, pregnant women, and any others who may not have a predictable heart rate response to cardiovascular exercise. In fact, RPE should probably be the preferred way to monitor exercise intensity in these types of situations. Make this decision after consultation with your qualified health care provider.

And finally, when RPE is used with heart rate monitoring, it provides a double check on the accuracy and effectiveness of your training heart rate (THR) zone. However, before you can use a THR, you need to be able to count your heart rate accurately.

Perceived Exertion Ratings: Borg's CR-10 Scale

0	Nothing at all	"No P"
0.3		
0.5	Extremely weak	Just noticeable
1	Very weak	
1.5		
2	Weak	Light
2.5		
3	Moderate	
4		
5	Strong	Heavy
6		
7	Very strong	
8		
9		
10	Extremely strong	"Max P"
11		
✦		
●	Absolute maximum	Highest possible

Borg CR10 scale
© Gunnar Borg, 1981, 1982, 1998

Measuring Heart Rate

Exercise heart rate or pulse is found by counting the number of times your heart beats in a minute. Counting the beats of your heart is pretty useless if it isn't done accurately or your THRR (training zone) is way off (more on this later). You can manually count your pulse at the wrist or use a heart rate monitor. There are pros and cons to both methods. Regardless, measuring heart rate is easy to do right.

Taking Your Pulse

One of the most practical and inexpensive ways to measure heart rate is using your fingertips to feel your pulse. The pulse of the heart is most often felt at the carotid artery (located on the front of the neck, and next to either side of the throat) and the radial artery at the wrist (located thumb side). The best location is near your wrist. To feel the radial pulse, place the index and middle finger lightly on the underside of the wrist. Don't use your thumb to monitor pulse, as it has a pulse of its own and may confuse you when counting.

KEY POINT

Inaccurate pulse counts result from starting the counts incorrectly, starting and ending on an incorrect time frame, improper hand placement, and miscounting the pulse during the timed pulse monitoring period.

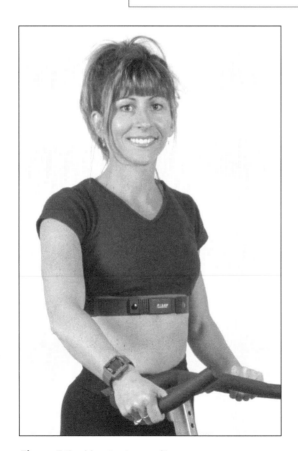

Figure 5.1 Heart rate monitor.

During activity, a 10-second heart rate count may be ideal. In a healthy person, exercise heart rate begins to slow quickly, usually after only 15 seconds, once exercise is stopped. It takes about two to four seconds to properly position finger placement to feel your pulse. By counting beats per 10 seconds, it is possible to complete the count within the crucial window of 15 seconds. This will avoid error as a result of heartbeat slowing down if longer counts are used and reflect your exercising heart rate.

Locate the pulse and repeatedly count "one, one, one..." to establish heart rate rhythm. Begin counting heart beats for 10 seconds when you've gotten a sense for the heartbeat pattern or rhythm. Remember to locate the pulse within seconds after exercise is completed or slowed.

For the 10-second count, start on a full beat as you pronounce "one." After counting heartbeats (pulses) during the 10 seconds, multiply by 6 to determine the heart rate in beats per minute.

If you've tried to feel your pulse and swear you don't have one, don't think you're crazy or completely incompetent. Even with correct technique, many people cannot feel their pulse. This may necessitate the use of a heart rate monitor. Additionally, research shows that most people are wildly inaccurate when counting their pulse. For example, some people say their heart rate is always 10 (for a 10-second count) because they count seconds rather than their pulse! This reality may help you reach the happy conclusion that the use of a heart rate monitor may be the easiest solution to accurate heart rate monitoring.

Using a Heart Rate Monitor

Using a heart rate monitor gives you immediate and accurate heart rates before, during, or after your workouts and only requires a quick glance at a watch. You don't have to stop, count, or calculate anything. This is good news for any of you who have ever crashed your bike or been shot off your treadmill while trying to take your pulse.

Wireless heart rate monitors are computerized, electronic digital readout devices that are designed to be worn on the wrist like a watch or mounted on exercise equipment. The heart rate monitor *constantly* displays your heart rate, giving you an updated heart rate every few seconds. Most include a clock, a timer, and an alarm that beeps when you're out of your training zone.

Accurate heart rate monitors transmit the electrical activity of the heart through an electrode harness or chest strap, much like you would find used during an ECG (electrocardiogram) in a doctor's office. The harness is positioned on the chest and sends the heart's electrical activity to a watchlike receiver mounted on exercise equipment or the wrist (see figure 5.1). The electrode transmits the heart rate, which is converted into a heart rate number that you read on the watch.

Because of occasional erroneous readings that may result from depleted batteries, product malfunctions, or other interferences, it is a good idea to use RPE or the talk test with heart rate monitors.

Finding Your Target Heart Rate (THR)

It's easy to figure out your THR (don't worry, this is not calculus). All you need to know is your resting and maximal heart rates. Resting heart rate (RHR) is found by counting your pulse for 60 seconds after waking in the morning. Do it several times over a one-week period. Maximal heart rate (MHR) is found by subtracting your age from 220, but you'll get a more accurate THR if you know your true MHR (more about that in a moment).

You should work between 40 and 85 percent of your reserve heart rate (HRR). If you're just starting a cardiovascular program, 40 to 60 percent is a realistic starting point. If you're in good shape, try 60 to 75 percent. If your cardiovascular system is really strong, 70 to 85 percent might work for your training range. Anaerobic interval training will require efforts that range from 85 to 100 percent of your HRR.

Using the Heart Rate Reserve Method

The heart rate reserve method (known as Karvonen's formula) is used to predict heart rate reserve (HRR). This method of calculating training zone accommodates various fitness level differences and more accurately predicts THR than other prediction methods because individual resting heart rate

(RHR) is entered into the formula. HRR is based on a simple concept. As you become more fit, your heart becomes stronger and more efficient so that for any given submaximal workload, heart rate will be lower. This includes resting heart rate. Using RHR to calculate your training ranges helps avoid lumping you into statistical averages, which can be less effective, inaccurate, and dangerous when calculating THRs.

It's tempting to use charts based on subtracting your age from 220 to predict MHR, and then taking a percentage of this predicted MHR to calculate a THR without taking into account RHR. Don't do it! This method leads to inaccurate heart rate training zones that are too easy or too hard. Remember, if you use 220 minus your age to predict MHR, you've already introduced a huge potential error component. At least the Karvonen formula considers RHR and gives you a somewhat more accurate picture.

The use of an *actual* MHR in the HRR equation is important, if possible. Maximal HR for 100 men aged 30 may vary from 166 to 214. Based on the age equation 220 minus 30, all of these individuals would have THRs predicted from an estimated MHR of 190 (their true MHR could be anywhere from 166 to 214!). The use of actual MHR and RHR in predicting THR in the Karvonen equation has profound implications in terms of personalizing training to your current fitness level.

Determining your actual or true MHR involves considerable motivation and is not advisable if you're not sure about your health. True MHR can easily be gotten by performing two to four minutes of all-out effort if peak heart rate is accurately monitored. A maximal aerobic capacity test or "max stress test" performed in a clinical setting is another way of determining actual MHR.

In order to use Karvonen's formula and calculate HRR, you must know your RHR, actual MHR, or predicted MHR (use 220 minus your age if you must). Use the work sheet on page 119. The example illustrates a prediction training heart rate (THR) for 80 percent, as estimated by the Karvonen formula.

To Monitor Heart Rate, or Not!

1. Heart rate may *not* be the best choice to monitor exercise intensity if you're taking medication. Check with your doctor to see if you should be using heart rate or RPE. In this scenario RPE is usually recommended unless you have a THRR (target heart rate range) that was prescribed while you were medicated. If this is the case, heart rate and RPE could be used together most effectively.

2. If you don't think you can accurately monitor HR, don't! If you're having trouble monitoring your pulse with your finger at your wrist, buy a heart rate monitor. With this assurance, you can trust your heart rate numbers.

3. Athletes and heart patients (in some instances) are examples of individuals who often require very accurate heart rate monitoring to optimize results or safety. As discussed, don't predict a THRR using the 220 minus your age formula, times a percentage. Be sure to predict your THRR (found by calculating an upper and lower limit THR) with the Karvonen formula. It is highly recommended that you use a reliable heart rate monitor rather than manual palpation.

Additionally, a normal heart rate response may not apply when swimming or participating in activities that use overhead arm movements, such as aerobic

Sample Calculation of THR Using the Karvonen Method

Maury is a 48-year-old man with a resting heart rate (RHR) of 79 who wishes to train at 80 percent of heart rate reserve (HRR). Here's how you calculate his THR using the Karvonen method:

1. Find Maury's estimated maximal heart rate (EMHR) using 220 – age since his true maximal heart rate (TMHR) is not available.

   EMHR = 220 – age

   EMHR = 220 – 48 = 172

2. Find Maury's heart rate reserve (HRR).

   HRR = (EMHR) – RHR

   HRR = _____172_____ (EMHR) – __79__ (RHR) = 93

3. Calculate Maury's target heart rate (THR).

   THR = HRR × training intensity % + RHR

   THR = __93__ (HRR) × _____.8_____ training intensity + __79__ (RHR)

   = HRR × percent training intensity + RHR

   = 74.4 + 79

   = 153.4 beats per minute (bpm)

   THR = 153 – 154 bpm (which is 80% of HRR plus RHR).

Worksheet for Calculating THR Using the Karvonen Method

The following worksheet allows you to calculate your target heart rate (THR) using either your true maximal heart rate (TMHR) as determined by a short, all-out effort (discussed previously) or your estimated maximal heart rate (EMHR) as determined by the formula 220 minus your age. You will recall from previous discussion that, when determining maximal heart rate (MHR), it is preferable to use a true rather than estimated or calculated MHR. Both resting heart rate and MHR numbers are necessary to calculate THR, using the Karvonen method.

1. Determine your resting heart rate (RHR) and your true maximal heart rate (TMHR) or estimated maximal heart rate (EMHR).

   Resting heart rate (RHR): _____

   True maximal heart rate (TMHR) or estimated maximal heart rate (EMHR): _____

2. Calculate heart rate reserve (HRR) using the following formula:

   (HRR) = (TMHR or EMHR)–RHR

   HRR = _____ (TMHR or EMHR) minus _____ (RHR)

   HRR = _____

3. Calculate target heart rate (THR) using the following formula:

   THR = HRR × training intensity % + RHR

   THR = ____ (HRR) × _____ (training intensity %) + _____ (RHR)

   THR = _____

   Or simply: THR = [MHR – RHR] × (training intensity %) + RHR

dance. That's why it's important to use the talk test and RPE in combination with heart rate.

What's The Perfect Effort?

Even though the talk test and RPE can stand alone as valid ways to ensure you're working at the right level of effort, heart rate gives an internal look at what is going on with your body. In theory, heart rate doesn't lie because it is an actual response of your body. It can tell you what kind of shape you're in, how much you've improved, and if you're training too hard. Heart rate is precise in its ability to tell you how your body is doing. It is an objective number rather than a subjective rating.

Having said that, combining the talk test, RPE, and heart rate measurement is the most precise way of gauging your level of effort. For example, if your training zone is slightly off and you're working at a heart rate that is too hard, using RPE or the talk test is going to tell you to back off. And if it's too easy, you know you can push a little harder.

Let's forget science, heart rate, and calculations for a minute. The golden rule with regard to gauging your level of effort is this: if it doesn't *feel* right, change your level of effort. Your preference for an exercise intensity and what you feel should dictate effort. A perfect effort that you will stick with will fall between some minimal range of not too hard or easy, in accordance with your training goals (obviously, anaerobic intervals are going to feel hard). In other words, exercise according to how you *feel*, rather than to a strict exercise heart rate which may not reflect a level of effort that is conducive to training result. What is most important is that you perceive your workouts as manageable and enjoyable, since such a wide range of exercise intensities confer health benefits. Approaching exercise with this attitude is safer and will promote long-term exercise compliance. And that's what it's all about, sticking to your exercise program, loving what you do, and getting results.

THE TOP AEROBIC EXERCISE

No one cardiovascular activity is better than another! Manipulating how hard, how often, and how long you perform a particular aerobic activity determines its effectiveness or lack thereof.

Choose the type of aerobic activity that is right for you by identifying an exercise that you can see yourself sticking to and enjoying for the rest of your life. If you discover an aerobic activity you are likely to do on a regular basis, then you've found a top cardiovascular activity.

Often, the best aerobic exercise will be not one, but several, activities that are fun, feel good to your body, keep your mind refreshed, and keep you progressing.

When cardiovascular fitness levels improve, your goals change, or your interests vary, you can use any large-muscle, rhythmic activity to keep your program on track. The final selection(s) depends on whether the cardiovascular activity fits you and whether you're motivated to pursue and stay with it. Excellent cardiovascular activities include, but are not limited to, walking, swimming, water fitness, jogging, running, cross-country skiing, in-line skating, lateral movement training (slide), cycling, mountain biking, and stair/step training.

As with all programming choices, don't take lightly your individual makeup and what drives you. Find activities that you love, look forward to, are passionate about, and truly enjoy. If you choose the right activity, you won't want to miss your workout for the world! You know you're on the right track when you guard your exercise time with the vigor of a lioness protecting newborn cubs!

Cardiovascular training does not have to be boring or repetitive or lead to overuse injuries. You can keep mentally and physically fresh by using several cardiovascular activities. Understanding how the energy systems interact will motivate you to change your workouts and intensity levels so you can fully develop your cardiovascular potential. And, by choosing workouts that enhance both the aerobic and anaerobic energy systems, you can keep cardiovascular conditioning interesting and results-oriented, regardless of your goals or current fitness level.

Quick Index:

6 Push Your Anaerobic Limits

Don't run from this chapter. Interval training can be for everyone. This especially holds true if you're looking for increased endurance/stamina, increased fat loss and calorie burning, and improved performance. Interval training will help you reach higher levels of fitness regardless of your current level of training or fitness.

What do an athlete in a competitive tennis match, a person running to the gate to catch an airplane, a person cross-country skiing over rolling terrain, an athlete performing bursts of intense activity in a team sport, and a grandmother climbing a hill during her afternoon walk have in common? All are using an effort interval, working a little harder than steady rate or what is comfortable. This acceleration in level of effort is then followed by a moderate recovery interval or time period in which activity returns to an easily sustainable level of effort. The beauty of an interval conditioning program is that the physiological requirements demanded of the body during interval conditioning are very similar to those needed for everyday life.

BENEFITS OF INTERVAL TRAINING

For many, interval training conjures up the terms *intense, hard*, and *painful,* and the image of professional athletes collapsing in an exhausted heap on the ground. Stay with me! Interval training can be done more moderately, too.

Why would you want to participate in interval training? Interval training can help you develop your cardiovascular system fully and maximize fat and calorie burning. It's fun, too, and helps to add variety to your cardiovascular training program. And you don't have to train like a pro athlete to get significant training benefits!

Interval conditioning can increase your ability to exercise longer at the limits of aerobic metabolism. This is greater than what can be accomplished with continuous training or aerobic training only. Because of this, interval training can help to improve fitness levels and total caloric expenditure.

Proper and appropriate interval conditioning can raise your anaerobic threshold whether you're deconditioned or very fit. This resultant change in anaerobic threshold allows you to work at increasingly more intense paces and for longer durations.

Overall, more total exercise effort is accumulated during an interval workout for a given time period. If you have limited time to exercise, this allows you to burn more total calories and fat and become more fit in a given exercise time period. Interval conditioning makes more effective use of your time whether you're deconditioned or highly fit.

Maximal oxygen uptake, or $\dot{V}O_2$ max (the most amount of oxygen your body can deliver and use to produce energy), along with the ability to sustain a high percentage of $\dot{V}O_2$ max, determines performance capabilities and your ability to optimize fitness gains. Anaerobic intervals increase your ability to sustain a higher percentage of $\dot{V}O_2$ max. This means you can work increasingly harder and longer and still maintain aerobic energy production. The highest level of effort that you can sustain aerobically is referred to as maximum steady rate (MSR). Increasing your anaerobic threshold or MSR is directly dependent on high-intensity anaerobic interval conditioning that is relative to your current fitness level.

KEY POINT

The use of interval conditioning has important implications for optimizing fitness gains, performance, interest, compliance, and results. Interval conditioning can optimize results whether you're highly trained or deconditioned. The key is to ensure that the training intensity is relative to your current state of fitness.

INS AND OUTS OF INTERVAL TRAINING

Optimizing cardiovascular conditioning requires that you work harder than an easy pace. Interval training involves short spurts of intensity harder than a comfortable level of effort (steady rate), followed by an easier intensity recovery effort (at or below steady rate).

Steady-Rate Pace

Interval training requires that you know what steady-rate pace is and feels like. Reviewing the information in chapter 5, steady-rate exercise is a level of cardiovascular effort that is easy to maintain. You might describe this level of intensity as aerobic or cruising, or characterize it by saying, I could keep this up all day long! Another good indicator of steady rate is whether or not you can sustain the pace for about two to three minutes or longer. If you're ready to crash and burn after 12 seconds, you're not working your muscles aerobically and are not at a steady rate of exercise.

Because you will be encouraged to work beyond this steady-rate comfort zone at times, such as during interval training efforts, it is important for you to understand how you feel during a steady-rate effort. Conversely, when you're recovering from vigorous interval exercise efforts, you will work at or below this level. Knowing what hard (above steady rate) or easy (below steady rate) exercise feels like will help optimize your interval training results. Both are equally important.

> ### KEY POINT
>
> Interval training or conditioning is simply working at a harder level of cardiovascular effort than what you are accustomed to. You do this by using intermittent work effort above your steady-rate level of effort and follow this with cardio activity that is steady rate or lower.

How Interval Training Works

Interval conditioning involves both aerobic and anaerobic processes. An important point to realize is that energy needs of the body's musculature are not switched on or off. Any time exercise intensity or duration changes, there will be an appropriate shift to either more or less involvement of a particular energy system, depending on the nature of the change. For example, as your cardiovascular workout lasts longer than about three minutes, the aerobic system supplies the largest percentage of the required energy to the working muscles. During high-intensity cardio activity up to about two to three minutes, anaerobic energy sources are the significant contributing factor.

For a healthy, untrained person, lactic acid begins to accumulate (the result of working above MSR and not being able to produce the required energy aerobically) and rises quickly at about 50 to 55 percent of maximal aerobic capacity, $\dot{V}O_2$ max, or heart rate reserve (HRR) (all of these terms mean essentially the same thing). If you're highly conditioned, this accumulation of lactic acid may not occur until 80 to 85 percent of HRR. (Calculating HRR is shown in chapter 5 and is of more practical use to you.)

At some point, whether at 50 percent, 85 percent, or some other percentage of HRR, you will reach a threshold, or a limiting factor, that does not allow you to continue performance at that particular level of intensity. This point of lactic acid accumulation is your anaerobic threshold.

Steady rate is a balance between energy demands of the muscle and aerobic metabolism. During steady-rate activity, any lactic acid production and accumulation is minimal.

Maximum steady-rate levels and anaerobic threshold vary from one individual to the next, depending primarily on a person's ability to deliver and use oxygen. This, of course, depends on individual genetics and conditioning level. For a sedentary person, going from rest to slow walking, let's say about 3 mph or a 20-minute-per-mile pace, may push his needs for energy (ATP) into anaerobic metabolism. In this case, maximum steady rate exists at very low intensity levels of activity. In contrast, the energy balance of a highly conditioned person can be maintained aerobically at very intense levels of exercise. For example, in a highly conditioned and genetically blessed marathon runner, steady-rate aerobic metabolism can be maintained at a pace near five-minutes-per-mile for 26 miles!

> **KEY POINT**
>
> Optimal cardiovascular fitness can only be realized by using both aerobic continuous training and anaerobic interval training.

MAXIMIZING FAT AND CALORIE BURNING

There is a lot of confusion surrounding the concept of fat burning versus carbohydrate burning. Should you slow down, go longer, or work harder to help you burn fat? Let's clear up a few fat myths.

Many people have been misled to believe that it is necessary to exercise for at least 20 minutes and work at a low exercise intensity to use fat. First, let's dispel the 20-minute myth. Even when you're flat on your back, the calories you burn come from *both* fat and carbohydrate. You are very aerobic at rest and therefore use fat. Clearly, it is *not* necessary to exercise a minimum of 20 minutes to begin using fat for energy. (Don't be discouraged if you can't last for 20 minutes. Something is better than nothing, and as you get stronger, you can eventually go longer.)

Do You Burn More Fat When You Go Slow?

The answer is yes and no, but mostly no. It is true that as you exercise *harder,* you burn a little *less* fat per calorie, and going *slower* burns a little *more* fat per calorie. This seems to support the idea that as exercise becomes harder, less *total* fat is burned. But this isn't the whole story. Cranking up the pace burns more total calories and more fat calories. That's because at the end of the harder workout you breathe more oxygen, which means you'll burn more calories and fat. Table 6.1 shows what this relationship looks like.

Table 6.1 Using Fat

Exercise intensity	Less intense: 30 minutes of exercise at 50% of heart rate reserve	More intense: 30 minutes of exercise at 75% of heart rate reserve
Result	More fat burned, about 50% from fat, per single calorie.	Less fat burned, about 40% from fat, per single calorie.
Total calories used	225	315
Total fat calories used	113	126

This data convincingly shows that for a given time period (30 minutes in this example), the harder pace of exercise burns more total fat and calories compared to a lesser intensity that burns more fat per single calorie.

What's the Best Level of Effort for Burning Fat and Losing Weight?

This whole discussion of burning fat and losing weight comes down to four key points:

1. Don't slow down or change how hard you're exercising if you can keep up the pace for however long you want to exercise. Exercising as hard as you comfortably can will *optimize* total calories and fat used. This type of continuous/aerobic training can also be alternated with low-level aerobic training. Both help you become more capable of burning fat.

2. If the exercise is too hard or cuts down on how long you'd like to exercise or your goal number of intervals, then it makes sense to slow down and go longer.

3. Working aerobically and anaerobically is necessary to optimize your ability to burn fat. Aerobic training has a different physiological impact than anaerobic training does, with regard to optimizing fat and calorie burning. That's why you need to do both.

4. To lose weight, most experts believe the key is the total number of calories you expend during exercise. Whether you're burning fat or carbohydrate does not seem to be important, so you don't even have to concern yourself with whether you're burning fat, or not!

Why Interval Training Maximizes Calories Burned

Many traditional workouts are designed to accommodate about 30 to 45 minutes of *continuous* cardiovascular training. If your goal is to lose weight, you'd be better off working at 80 percent of your $\dot{V}O_2$ max or HRR. However, even though 80 percent of HRR would maximize calorie and fat utilization compared to a lesser level of intensity, it is a much more difficult workout. A more realistic exertion level would be about 70 percent of HRR, if you're fairly fit. This intensity level is more likely to be maintained over 30 to 45 minutes, and this level of effort still uses plenty of calories.

But, if you have difficulty maintaining high or even moderate levels of continuous cardiovascular effort, interval conditioning allows you to accumulate more total exercise performed at higher intensities and in tolerable doses of duration. Many people find it much easier to endure relatively short durations of higher-intensity work. And these higher intensities will eventually allow you to work at higher levels of effort in relative comfort. Previously, this same effort would have exhausted you quickly.

If you are deconditioned, you should probably exercise at a level of intensity you can maintain to optimize fat and calorie burning. Build your base of conditioning with moderate levels of effort that last three or more minutes and worry about optimizing how hard you work as you become more fit. As your fitness improves, work out at manageable effort intervals of slightly higher intensity than that to which you're accustomed, in addition to your regular aerobic training.

TOP INTERVAL TRAINING MODELS

Interval training design may be more art (read this as "experience, trial and error, and observing what works") than science. But, you can't find a better starting point to begin or enhance your current interval training program than speed play and the following health and fitness interval and performance interval training models. But first, it's important to lay the groundwork for these top training recipes.

Interval Training Concepts and Terminology

Interval conditioning uses repeated cardiovascular effort intervals that are performed above intensities that you're used to working at, such as that which occurs during steady-rate effort or continuous training. In order to sustain and repeat these higher intensities, the effort intervals are followed by cardiovascular recovery intervals that are performed at a steady rate or lower intensity. An effort interval followed by a recovery interval is termed a cycle.

Aerobic interval conditioning involves training just below, at, or slightly above lactate or maximum steady-rate (MSR) threshold. Although some anaerobic metabolism occurs to supply the energy need in this type of effort, especially if above MSR, it is predominantly aerobic.

On the other hand, anaerobic interval conditioning involves training significantly *above*, and recovering at or below, anaerobic or MSR threshold. This type of training requires a predominance of anaerobic energy metabolism.

Speed Play

If you're in good shape, or not-so-great shape, or have never tried interval training, you may want to begin with speed play. It's easy to experiment with speed play. In this type of training you increase cardiovascular effort for various amounts of time and follow this with adequate recovery. For example, if you're running, cycling, or walking outdoors, you might speed up a little until you reach a stop sign that is several hundred yards away. This 30 seconds or so of effort is followed by three times more rest, or 90 seconds of easy recovery. You can "play" as many times as you like, and you choose the intensity.

> ### KEY POINT
> Speed play works whether you're highly fit or deconditioned because you can keep the training intensity relative to your current fitness level.

Health and Fitness Interval Training Model

Health and fitness intervals have a broad and clear application to most people. This type of interval training is more structured than speed play intervals and can be performed using an aerobic or an anaerobic model. The goal is to work from "somewhat hard" to "very hard" on the RPE scale. Aerobic intervals have you work from "somewhat hard" to "hard" for two to three minutes. This is followed by the same amount of recovery. If you pick up your pace for two minutes, you recover for two minutes. During anaerobic intervals you work a little harder, "hard" to "very hard," but for only 30 to 90 seconds. You also recover for three times the time spent working at a harder pace. If you pick it up for 30 seconds, you recover for 90 seconds. During recovery you should reach a level that feels easy before you go for another interval. Doing about five or six effort/recovery intervals (cycles) is adequate, but most important, go by how you feel.

Intensity is controlled by you. The key is to simply work at a pace a little harder than that to which you are accustomed. This approach allows you to select an individualized exercise intensity while the length (duration) of each interval is set.

KEY POINT

An important advantage interval conditioning has over continuous training is that it can challenge *both* the aerobic and anaerobic systems. This, of course, leads to optimal cardiovascular conditioning. Proper intensity and duration must be observed to effectively achieve this goal.

Experts recommend a 1:1 effort-to-recovery ratio in aerobic fitness intervals. In scientific literature this ratio is referred to as the work-to-rest ratio. This ratio implies that there is an equal amount of effort to recovery in each interval cycle. It does *not* mean that one minute of effort is always followed by one minute of recovery. For example, using a 1:1 effort-to-recovery ratio, a three-minute effort interval is followed by a three-minute recovery interval.

During anaerobic fitness intervals a 1:3 effort-to-recovery ratio is used. Using this ratio, a one-minute effort interval will be followed by a three-minute recovery interval. Generally, it is best to perform anaerobic effort intervals for a duration of 90 seconds or less. If effort intervals are performed at proper intensity, a 90-second or less duration ensures that the anaerobic system will receive a conditioning challenge.

Because you determine your own level of exertion, and the effort should remain moderate (steady rate), it is *not* necessary that you have a high level of fitness to participate in aerobic intervals. Relative to current level of fitness, it's easy for anyone to work a little harder than normal. However, the *anaerobic* fitness interval model that follows does assume a moderate to high level of fitness.

In either model, intensity is ultimately determined by you, but you are encouraged to push your level of effort so that it corresponds to the recommended RPE rating (see table 6.2, Interval Training Summary, page 133). Everyone's perception will be different, but the end goal would be to work the interval at a level of effort that is higher than what you would normally do and corresponds to the descriptive ratings (i.e., "somewhat hard" to "hard"). Think of the specific RPE guidelines as your personal trainer, encouraging you on to greater efforts and results. (Note: If you choose to follow the performance interval model, in which exercise intensity is predetermined, you'll be encouraged to use RPE and/or heart rate to monitor effort and recovery intervals.)

Aerobic Fitness Model

Ratio: 1:1 effort-to-recovery (work-to-rest ratio)

Duration: 3–5 minutes for effort interval

3–5 minutes for recovery interval

Minutes of effort/recovery may vary from 3 to 5 minutes as long as the 1:1 ratio of effort to recovery is observed for each cycle.

Intensity: Participant controlled

Effort intervals: 4–6 on RPE scale

Recovery intervals: 2–3 on RPE scale

Frequency: Number of cycles accomplished depends on time availability and your fitness level and goals.

Anaerobic Fitness Model

Ratio: 1:3 effort-to-recovery

Duration: 30–90 seconds for effort interval

1.5–4.5 minutes for recovery interval

Duration of effort and recovery can vary within the above parameters as long as the 1:3 ratio of effort to recovery is observed for each cycle.

Intensity: Participant controlled

Effort intervals: 7–10 on RPE scale

Recovery intervals: 2–3 on RPE scale

Frequency: Number of cycles accomplished depends on time availability and your fitness level and goals.

Performance Interval Training Model

You might be a competitive triathlete, race-walker, or runner wanting to increase your speed. Or, you might be superbly conditioned, a little bored, looking for a challenge and more results, and wanting to take your level of cardiovascular fitness to the next level. Performance intervals are an excellent training technique to enhance higher levels of cardiovascular fitness and performance.

The most structured of the interval formulas, this particular model for performance intervals is an example of classic, high-intensity performance interval training. Before you use it, make sure you're highly conditioned, properly motivated, and ready to train in a structured and physically intense environment.

Performance intervals require the use of precise, high-intensity work periods interspersed with specific recovery periods. Training focus is on *intensity* of effort for specific effort intervals and durations. Effort and recovery intervals should not be randomly manipulated if specific performance training goals have been identified and are desired. To follow these guidelines, you must be highly fit and extremely motivated.

During performance intervals, heart rate monitoring with a wireless heart rate monitor is recommended. Perceived exertion (RPE) works well if you understand the relationship between heart rate response and RPE, but this relationship needs to be established through accurate heart rate monitoring that is associated with an RPE.

The three performance interval models that follow assume a high level of fitness.

Intensity, duration, and frequency are *fixed* according to specific performance goals. Use RPE and heart rate to monitor effort and recovery intervals; monitor heart rate with an electronic heart rate monitor. Notice that there are two anaerobic performance interval models. The second continues to challenge you as your cardiovascular fitness level progresses. Model #2 not only increases exercise intensity, but also simultaneously decreases recovery time, which makes the interval very challenging.

Aerobic Performance Model

Ratio: 1:1 effort-to-recovery

Duration: 3–5 minutes for effort interval

3–5 minutes for recovery interval

Duration of effort and recovery can vary within the above parameters as long as the 1:1 ratio of effort to recovery is observed for each cycle.

Intensity: Fixed

Effort intervals: 80–85% of HRR (4–6 on RPE scale)

Recovery intervals: 2–3 on RPE scale

Frequency: Number of cycles accomplished depends on time availability and your fitness level/goals.

Anaerobic Performance Model #1

Ratio: 1:3 effort-to-recovery

Duration: 30–90 seconds for effort interval

90–270 seconds (1.5–4.5 minutes) for recovery interval

Duration of effort and recovery can vary within the above parameters as long as the 1:3 ratio of effort to recovery is observed for each cycle.

Intensity: Fixed

Effort intervals: 85–90% of HRR (5–8 on RPE scale)

Recovery intervals: 2–3 on RPE scale

Frequency: Number of cycles accomplished depends on time availability and your fitness level/goals.

Anaerobic Performance Model #2

Ratio: 1:2 effort-to-recovery

Duration: 30–90 seconds for effort interval

60–180 seconds (1–3 minutes) for recovery interval

Duration of effort and recovery can vary within the above parameters as long as the 1:2 ratio of effort to recovery is observed for each cycle.

Intensity: Fixed

Effort intervals: Greater than 90% of HRR (8–10 on RPE scale)

Recovery intervals: 2–3 on RPE scale

Frequency: Number of cycles accomplished depends on time availability and your fitness level/goals.

Recovery After Interval Training Efforts

Anaerobic interval conditioning is performed at the expense of lactic acid buildup in the exercising muscles and blood. Recovery from anaerobic intervals takes longer and is reflected by the ratios of effort and recovery durations.

Recovery of proper duration and intensity after anaerobic effort intervals is crucial. It is during recovery that many of the specific training adaptations occur. In other words, many of the benefits and training results you earn from your interval training come during recovery. Don't cut it short. It is as important as the effort!

In addition, active recovery helps speed your recovery from your interval efforts. In active recovery, submaximal exercise (usually steady rate or lower) is performed in the belief that this continued movement prevents muscle cramps and stiffness and facilitates the recovery process.

Lactic acid removal is accelerated by active recovery exercise and clearly is more effective in facilitating lactic acid removal than passive recovery (i.e., lying down). Easy aerobic exercise may facilitate the removal of lactic acid because of increased blood flow. Increased availability of blood flow and oxygen to the muscle, at moderate levels of exercise, would allow the lactic acid to be used within the muscle.

KEY POINT

Low-level, active recovery will be the rule for interval recoveries. During recovery intervals, maintain an intensity of steady rate or lower and a duration that equals or exceeds the effort interval duration. Active recovery is of great importance when recovering from intervals that produce appreciable levels of lactic acid and for maximizing training results.

Probably, if left to your own intuition, you'll naturally select an optimal-recovery exercise intensity. This will be at one of the following levels:

1. Just below your lactic acid accumulation threshold; in other words, at a level of exercise intensity that you can easily maintain

2. Where you're not breathless and can speak three or four words at a time without gasping

3. Where your muscles are not burning or uncomfortable from lactic acid accumulation

4. A "somewhat easy" or "moderate" level of exertion, which rates 2 to 3 on the RPE scale

Table 6.2 provides a summary of the relationships between RPE, HRR, and RPE descriptive ratings. Corresponding intensity-level categories and sample activities are also included.

Aerobic, and especially anaerobic, interval intensities can represent levels of intensity to which you are not accustomed. You should probably have a moderate level of fitness to do aerobic intervals and a high-level fitness base (at least four to six weeks of progressive aerobic training) to participate in anaerobic interval conditioning.

The RPE scale recommends a 2 to 3 level of effort (40 to 60 percent of HRR) for warm-up, cool-down, and recovery from your effort intervals. Aerobic intervals require a 4 to 5 (80 to 85 percent of HRR) or 5 to 7 (85 to 90 percent of HRR) level of effort, and anaerobic interval training will push you toward a 100 percent effort. Remember that athletes require precise intensities, depending on their performance goals. However, the key to developing your anaerobic conditioning with less precise methods is to regularly work harder than you are used to working. Effective interval training can be that simple!

Guidelines for Performing Intervals Safely and Effectively

1. As with any type of fitness activity, precede the intervals with a warm-up of at least 5 to 10 minutes and follow it with a cool-down of at least 5 minutes. After the cool-down you should feel that your heart rate and breathing are back to pre-exercise levels.

2. If you feel ready for the next interval, then do it. If you need more time to recover, take it. Remember, common sense always rules, even if you're following one of the interval models that specifies the amount of recovery. A guideline is just that, a guideline. Keep interval training fun, challenging, and aligned with your workout goals.

3. Beginning or deconditioned exercisers should not participate in interval conditioning that pushes to an RPE of 7 to 10 ("very hard" to "very, very hard").

4. Carefully monitor your exertion level. Exhaustion is not the goal. Interval training should be enjoyable and, though challenging, should not create lingering exhaustion or a negative experience.

5. Remember, how hard you push is controlled by you, even though you are encouraged to go beyond your comfort zone.

6. Interval training workouts that repeat about 10 to 12 anaerobic efforts should be used only once or twice per week. Monitor your workouts and get enough rest to avoid overtraining.

Table 6.2 Interval Training Summary

Intensity level categories	RPE	%HRR	RPE descriptive rating (How the exercise feels)	Examples of activities
"Lounging around"	0–1	Very low	"Very, very easy"	Channel surfing
Warm-up Low-level activity Recovery	2–3	40–60	"Somewhat easy" to "Moderate"	An easy walk, run, aerobic cool-down, or recovery after an interval
Steady rate	3–4	40–80	"Moderate" to "Somewhat hard"	A sustained, but manageable aerobic workout
Aerobic interval effort	4–5 5–7	80–85 85–90	"Hard" to "Very hard"	Cardio effort that lasts up to 3 minutes
Anaerobic interval effort	7–8 9–10	90–95 95–100+	"Very hard" to "Very, very hard" or "That's it!"	Cardio effort that lasts up to 90 seconds

Quick Index:

Lift for Strength and Muscle Definition

After reading this chapter you won't ever be confused by much-hyped terms such as *muscle tone*, *body shaping*, *lifting to get cut*, or *defined*; concepts such as using special equipment to build "long, lean muscles" (you can't!); and the differences between muscular endurance and strength. Plus, you'll know how to design strength training programs (or you can follow the ones I give you) that are time-efficient and help you attain your strength training goals.

WHAT STRENGTH TRAINING IS, AND ISN'T

What's the difference between resistance training, strength training, weight lifting, weight training, lifting weights, and pumping iron? No wonder everyone's confused. There really is none. Choose your favorite term and stick with it (or if you want to impress your friends or confuse them too, use all of them).

Working against resistance—for example, lifting a dumbbell or handheld weight a number of times or pulling on rubber tubing—is commonly referred to as resistance training. The term *resistance training* is an umbrella term used to cover *all* types of strength or weight training.

Resistance training includes free weights (such as dumbbells, barbells, handheld weights, and freeplates, which are those metal discs that slide onto long or short bars and if not attached properly fall on your feet or head), elastic resistance, weight machines, and even your own body weight (e.g., when you do a push-up). Weight doesn't have to come in the form of a rock or dumbbell. Tubing works great, too.

I use the terms *resistance training* and *strength training* most of the time, but regardless, I know you won't be confused again by this array of terminology.

BENEFITS OF STRENGTH TRAINING

Strength training not only develops muscular strength and muscular endurance and improves performance, but it can also help your muscles recover from the daily physical stresses of life and change how you look. Additionally, physical fitness declines with age. However, many of the detrimental changes in physiological function are due to decreased physical activity and the resultant muscle loss that often accompany aging. Strength training increases and preserves muscle, which minimizes the negative, age-related changes in physiological function (many of which are described in the box on page 137). The following sections outline five good reasons to strength train.

> **KEY POINT**
>
> The so-called inevitable decline in personal health with age results largely from muscle loss and can be prevented to a large degree with a regular strength training program. Strength training twice per week can avoid a cascade of negative health consequences.

Lose Fat and Control Your Weight

Because it can increase your metabolism, strength training may be the most important exercise you can do for losing fat and maintaining your weight. Now, don't throw away your running and walking shoes just yet. Even though biking, running, and dance aerobics do not develop muscle to any great extent, aerobic training is still important for health and weight control. Nevertheless, one of the biggest reasons people gain weight is that they lose muscle.

Metabolism refers to the number of calories you're burning whether sleeping, watching TV, or exercising vigorously. Metabolism slows with age, but the bulk of the decrease has nothing to do with getting older. It seems to be caused mostly by physical inactivity. You can lose 1 percent of your muscle annually if you don't exercise, which means from the age of 30 until the age of 75 you can lose 45 percent of your muscle! If you do only aerobics such as running, walking, and biking, you will lose muscle over time. The key to avoiding muscle loss is to strength train!

Increase muscle and you'll burn more calories naturally—24 hours per day—even at rest. This will help you *lose* fat and *maintain* your desired weight.

You burn calories during and after lifting, but strength training also increases your metabolism (the rate at which you burn calories) at rest because it causes an increase in muscle mass. Muscle tissue is very metabolically active. (Muscle is like Pac-Man; it gobbles up lots of calories to maintain itself, unlike fat which requires almost no calories to exist.) Muscle makes you a calorie waster, which means it burns calories so they won't be stored as fat. Bottom line: Increasing or maintaining muscle will help you burn more calories and keep the fat off!

Improve Your Personal Appearance

All of us would like to be pleased with what we see in the mirror. Regardless of how you *think* you look, self-acceptance is important.

Strength training does some good things for your image that aerobics can't. It shapes, strengthens, builds, and develops muscle. This has a direct impact on how you look. For example, your padded shoulders are now the result of muscles being developed instead of pieces of foam stuffed in your blouse; a caved-in chest now looks strong, full, and expanded; and your sleeveless dress shows off tone where "flappies of fat" used to hang from the back of your arms. Though you can't spot-*reduce*, or selectively cause fat to disappear from a particular body part, you can spot-*tone*. And, if you shape up a particular body part, eat right, and do aerobic exercise, you'll lose fat and look strong!

Get Stronger and Reduce Your Risk of Injury

Strong muscles will make you less likely to get hurt. With strong muscles come strong ligaments (they support your joints) and strong tendons (they connect muscles to bone). What this means is that you have margin for error. For example, if you stumble or lose your balance, there's a good chance you can right yourself without falling or hurting yourself.

Have Strong, Healthy Bones

Millions of Americans have osteoporosis, which is a disease that cripples by weakening bones. This can lead to fractures in the hip, back, and wrist. Fracture complications can result in complete inactivity and an astonishing decrease in personal well-being. And don't think you have to fall to break a weak bone. A quick turn of the head can break a vertebrae, or catching your balance after a slip can fracture your hip. Strong bones are solid and dense, like a strong slab of oak. Diseased bones look like porous sponges and break easily when stressed, like wood diseased with dry rot.

But isn't osteoporosis a disease of the frail and elderly? Let's get this straight. Osteoporosis *can* contribute to making a *healthy* older person frail, weak, and sick. However, it is a disease of the young. It starts early in life and is a killer because you don't know you have it until it's difficult to reverse the damage. The key to preventing osteoporosis is to maintain the bone you have. Good nutrition and exercise are the keys, starting in the teen years. Even if you're well beyond this youthful age, you can still build some bone back by strength training and participating in weight-bearing aerobic exercise such as walking. Proper intake of calcium and vitamin D are also important.

Strong muscles mean strong bones. When you contract your muscles by lifting weights, the point at which the muscles attach to the bone are positively stressed. These attachment points actually pull on the bone. This is what keeps your bones strong (don't forget good nutrition). That is why complete inactivity contributes to weak and unhealthy bones.

Stay Healthy

Strength training can lower your blood pressure if it's high and reduce your risk for diabetes and some types of cancer. It can also lower your risk for heart disease by increasing good cholesterol and decreasing bad cholesterol.

Health Benefits Associated With Resistance Training

(If you don't strength train, turn each one of these benefits around 180 degrees and see the consequence!)

Fat loss, weight control, weight maintenance. Losing weight is the wrong goal. You can lose the wrong kind of weight (muscle and bone) and still be fat. Focus on dropping fat and gaining muscle.

Increased metabolism. If you have a lot of muscle, your metabolism is higher and you need more calories since muscle is metabolically active.

Increased calorie burning during resistance training.

Increased calorie burning after exercise.

Reductions in resting blood pressure. If you have high blood pressure or borderline high blood pressure, use moderate loads and 15 to 20 repetitions. You can lower your blood pressure by decreasing the amount of salt and alcohol in your diet, losing weight, and exercising.

Decreased risk for diabetes. Diabetes ultimately results from an inability to control blood sugar levels. Insulin that is secreted from your pancreas normally controls blood sugar levels. Muscle tissue is programmed to respond to insulin and, as ordered by this hormone, to take sugar out of the blood into the muscle. As people get fatter, older, and inactive, the muscle tissue they have left doesn't obey insulin command orders. Solution: lift weights, build muscle, and lose fat!

Positive changes in blood lipid profiles. HDL cholesterol (the good guy) is raised only by exercise (aerobic and strength training) and losing fat. Of course, diet is important to lower harmful LDL (the bad guy) and triglycerides.

Decreased risk for osteoporosis and increased bone mineral content. You can avoid weaker, less dense, and more brittle bone by strength training and using weight-bearing exercise (e.g., walking and running). You'll be at less risk for fracture resulting from inactivity if you maintain weight-bearing aerobic and strength training throughout your life.

Improved structural and functional integrity of tendons, ligaments, and joints.

Thicker and stronger tendons (which connect muscles to bones) **and ligaments** (which provide integrity to joints by connecting bone to bone). Stronger muscles let you exert more force and perform better with less chance of injury to the muscles, tendons, ligaments, and joints.

Personal physical independence. Many people lose their freedom because they've lost the strength to be mobile.

Enhanced physical activity experiences. Strong individuals perform better, and physical activity feels good to their bodies.

Improved posture. Strength and flexibility are the keys to correct body alignment.

Improved physical image. Strength training will change how you look. If you don't believe this, take a look at a runner who only trains the cardiovascular system.

Improved self-esteem. You'll feel strong, look strong, and think that you're strong!

PUTTING STRENGTH TRAINING MYTHS TO REST

The many misconceptions about strength training are like weeds that spread through your yard and won't go away. Everyone has some idea of what they *think* happens when weights are lifted, but are these impressions accurate? In the next few sections I'll answer some common strength training questions—with the facts.

Will I Get Big, Bulky Muscles If I Strength Train?

Maybe, and maybe not! Around puberty (you remember that disastrous time that occurs near the ages of 12 to 14) boys and girls are at similar strength levels. Males gain a strength advantage when they enter puberty because their bodies start to crank up the production of the predominantly male-dominant hormone testosterone. Men have levels that are 20 to 30 times higher than women, which makes it easier for them to build more muscle. While some women possess high levels of this hormone, most don't, which is part of the reason that you see fewer women who do in fact build big muscles.

This is only one component that determines the size of muscles, however. Illegal drugs and genetics are the other two important factors. Many of the oversized men and women on the pump-you-up shows are taking drugs that allow them to develop physiques that truly make you wonder if they come from another planet. This is not natural, safe, ethical, or normal!

The type and amount of muscle you have, along with body type (i.e., thin, round, strong, or stout), are determined by your parents. In other words, your genetics greatly influence the results you'll see from any type of strength training program. For example, if you have a small, wiry body you'll see some great strength improvements, but you'll probably never be bulging with muscles.

Is It Easier for Some People to Build Muscle and Get Stronger?

Yes. Some people are genetically blessed with regard to developing strength and muscle. Two people (same gender and similar body types) could participate in the same program and end up with completely different results. Sometimes it doesn't seem quite fair when two people invest the same effort and time and one seems to get better results. This is what I refer to as the reality factor; scientists call it individual response.

Here's a positive way of looking at it. Don't compare yourself to others. Look at where you started and how far you've come in terms of your fitness. You can improve 100 percent when compared to *your* starting point, so keep your focus on personal improvements.

Since the outer bounds of your personal fitness are genetically determined (you have no influence even though you'd like to look like Rambo or Ramboette), there is a lot of truth to the statement, Champion athletes are born. Fortunately, your health and personal fitness have nothing to do with being "numero uno" or "body perfect."

Do Some Machines or Kinds of Weight Equipment Develop Long, Lean Muscles?

No! This claim is so far from the truth it's hard to figure where it came from. Genetics, how much resistance you work against, and how often you train are the biggest contributors to how your muscles develop.

How Long Before I Feel Stronger and See Changes?

Men and women of all ages (even 70, 80, and 90 years young!) can increase their strength by more than 50 percent just two months after beginning a strength training program. If you keep training, you can double, or even triple, your strength!

Many people who start lifting experience immediate changes in terms of balance, coordination, and strength. Technically speaking, initial strength improvements that happen in the first four to six weeks of your strength program happen because you get more skillful. This means that you learn how to lift better. During these first few weeks, changes also occur in the nerves (nervous system) that help you use muscle that was "sleeping," or inactive, before you started pumping weight.

> ### KEY POINT
> Runners, cyclists, walkers: Even though your heart is strong, you need to strength train!

Physical changes in the muscle start after about six weeks. This is called hypertrophy, which means an increased muscle size. Most people believe big muscles are strong muscles. To a certain degree that is true, but remember that you can get strong without seeing your muscles change.

Moreover, "humongo" muscles don't necessarily translate well to everyday tasks that involve coordination and balance. Don't measure muscle strength by size alone! You have to ask, Is this functional strength, or in other words, useable?

What Happens to My Muscles When I Get Stronger?

As already mentioned, most (almost 80 percent) of the strength gains you'll get come from your nerves being able to rally dormant muscle fibers to contract and move the body. The other 20 percent or so comes from your muscles getting bigger (hypertrophy). The role that your nerves play explains why some people keep getting stronger without getting bigger muscles.

What about bulking up? Quite honestly, most people have difficulty putting large amounts of muscle on their body. Certain body types are more likely to develop muscle than others. For example, if you're thin (everyone has been calling you "String-bean" for years), there's a good chance you won't develop big muscles even though you'll get stronger and more defined and your running will improve. If you've been nicknamed "Refrigerator" for more years than you'd like to remember, you're a good candidate for the sport of body building, but don't forget cardiovascular training and developing a strong, healthy heart.

And, *nothing* positive will happen to your muscles if you don't use enough weight or resistance in the form of tubes, body weight, machines, or dumbbells. Little will happen with regard to increased muscle size or strength gains if you use light weights and high repetitions (more on this later). On the other hand, if you slough off and don't weight train, your muscles will shrink. This is called atrophy. You've heard it before—use it or lose it!

How Do I Get Muscle Definition?

Genetics, what you were sentenced to at birth, may be the most important factor in gaining muscle definition. However, the two steps you can take to influence muscle definition are to lose fat and strength train.

Do My Muscles Turn to Fat if I Stop Strength Training?

No, no, no, no! Under a microscope fat looks like Honeycomb cereal and muscle like a bundle of straws. The point is, they are *different* from one another.

The misconception that muscle turns to fat may have started because many highly trained athletes have become fat after their sport careers ended. Here's the real picture. The athlete quit training; the muscles shrank; and the athlete continued to slop down the grits, bacon, steaks, and beer, or at least took in too many calories. The extra calories were stored as fat. The only way muscles can grow is by being challenged by strength training!

Does Strength Training Spot-Reduce Problem Areas?

Strength training, or for that matter any exercise, has nothing to do with spot-reducing. Spot-reduction is *not* possible. You lose fat when you burn off more calories than you take in. This can be accomplished by exercising (cardiovascular and strength training is the best approach) and moderate calorie reduction. Even though you may chew on your TV remote or vigorously chomp on gum, this does not reduce flapping jowls or double chins. Spot-reduction sounded too good to be true anyway.

Should I Get in Shape Before I Start Lifting Weights?

This is one of the biggest *myth*-conceptions of all and deters many people who should be lifting weights. Just to make sure this registers, the answer is no! People who are extremely overweight often begin a strength training program *before* aerobics! Why? Increased strength may help protect joints from injury and improve aerobic activity that requires lower body strength. Lifting weights is nonimpact, and increased muscle gained from lifting can help burn more calories, facilitate weight loss, and increase metabolism. Besides, it's fun, interesting, and keeps you motivated since it's a lot more gratifying than *only* doing endless miles on a treadmill!

Do I Have to Spend Hours Training to Get Results?

It's not a requirement that you sentence yourself to four to six hours in the gym laboring over weights, divorce your spouse, and forget about your kids to receive benefits from strength training. I'll talk more on this later, but here's the minimal commitment: Strength train twice a week for about 20 minutes per workout. That's it? you say. Yes, and no strings attached. Now, I've just retired your last reason for not strength training—that you don't have the time. If you're not pumping, it's time to start!

Should a Woman's Strength Program Differ From a Man's?

It is NOT true that a woman's strength training program should differ from a man's. Some books written for women infer that women need to train differently. Sorry. Not true. No physiologist has ever discovered a female or male muscle fiber, and correct technique does not change from gender to gender. There are simply muscle fibers and a right way to perform exercises, regardless of gender. When women are placed on the same strength programs men are using, they make the same, if not greater, gains in muscle strength and endurance. Men and women are different. But the quality of a woman's muscle fiber compares to that of a man's, although she may have less (quantity) and may not have as strong an influence from the muscle-building hormone testosterone. These influences aside, men and women should not train differently. Personal and sport-oriented goals should dictate how the individual should train, independent of being male or female.

PLANNING YOUR STRENGTH PROGRAM

There are literally hundreds of strength programs you could follow. Are any of these programs really that different from one another? Are they safe and effective and do they produce results in a time-efficient manner? The answer to these two questions is, more often than not, no and probably not.

Different strength programs are lumped under the term *systems*. A system is any combination of reps, number of sets, and weight you work against that some "yahoo" has given a name. Often the system's driving force is some kind of hype that sells useless products or services, and it usually doesn't stick around for long. Remember, anyone can name a system and popularize some idiotic approach to strength training that will eventually disgust you, hurt you, and frustrate you. (As you may sense, I feel strongly about this particular discussion.) Some of the dumbest programs carry names such as the 100-Rep System and Pump Until You Puke. These types of systems have nothing to do with sensible training that will yield results.

The following sections outline what you need to know about your strength training program. Once this foundation of knowledge is laid, you can accomplish your strength training goals safely and in the least amount of time.

Amount of Weight (or Resistance)

People often ask how much weight they should use. It's the wrong question, but the right idea! It is not how much weight you lift that is the key, but the number of repetitions you perform. Just the number of reps? Well, yes, kind of. What you need to do is work within a specific framework or number of reps until your muscles are tired.

Starting Weight

If you're just starting a strength program, it's important not to test your ability to lift the most amount of weight you can for a given lift. This is called a 1-RM or 1-repetition max. If you're just starting, don't put yourself in a high-risk, maximal-performance situation. Err on the side of using too little weight rather than too much to determine starting points. For example, if you're doing more reps than you've set for your repetition parameters, you can easily bring the number of reps down by increasing resistance.

> ### KEY POINT
>
> The starting load is determined by an appropriate resistance that fatigues the muscle within the stated repetition goal range.

Number of Repetitions

"Rep" is gym slang for "repetition." You count reps by counting the number of times you complete a strength exercise by returning to the start position. Ninety-nine percent of the American population should be doing 6 to 20 reps to fatigue.

If you're new to strength training, you might be asking, What's this fatigue stuff? Some people refer to this as muscle failure. Fatigue is the point somewhere between 6 and 20 reps at which you can't do another repetition with good form. It is not necessary to motivate or psych yourself to squeeze out one more rep because you've heard that it's the last one that really counts. *Not* true!

Should everyone work to fatigue? I know this can be a threatening concept, but the answer is yes—everyone. Now, if you're just starting or out of shape, the number of reps to fatigue that you should complete should fall between 15 and 20, but it's better to shoot for 20 initially. This number will give your muscles, tendons, and ligaments a chance to get in shape and prevent you from doing too much too soon. If you've been training four to six weeks at 15 to 20 reps, you may want to aim for 12 to 15 reps to see continued and significant changes in strength and muscle size. To maximize your strength and muscle size gains, drop down to 6 to 12 (see table 7.1). You'll have to increase the weight you're lifting to drop down to this lower number of reps. (After you've trained consistently for about six months, you'll periodize your program to periodically work, once again, in all three rep ranges. See chapters 2 and 11.)

Muscular strength and endurance conditioning is anaerobic work that should last only about 30 to 90 seconds; the targeted muscles should fatigue

Table 7.1 What You Need To Know About Reps and Intensity

Number of reps	What you get!	How hard?	When?
15–20	Muscle endurance, strength, tone, and health benefits	Enough resistance to cause muscle fatigue between 15 and 20 reps	First 4–6 weeks of training even if you're just starting or out of shape, regardless of age
12–15	Muscle endurance, strength, size, and health benefits	Enough resistance to cause muscle fatigue between 12 and 15 reps	After 4–6 weeks of training at 15–20 reps, if you want to continue to significantly progress your strength program
6–12	Maximum muscle strength and size (hypertrophy) and health benefits	Enough resistance to cause muscle fatigue between 6 and 12 reps	After 4–6 weeks of training at 12–15 reps to fatigue to maximize strength and muscle size

or fail within this time frame. Generally, 6 to 20 repetitions performed in a controlled manner will fit into this time parameter and produce significant strength gains.

Let's go back to the question of how much weight. Remember, wrong question! Pick enough resistance to fatigue your muscles in one of these three repetition frameworks. Regardless of whether the goal is 15 to 20, 12 to 15 or 6 to 12 reps, you'll find people of different strengths will have to work with *different* amounts of weight or resistance to optimize their personal training results. Consider, for example, two people performing an arm (biceps) curl side by side. While both fatigue at 15 reps, one is using a 25-pound weight and the other is using an 8-pound weight. Nevertheless, both will see significant gains in strength and are working at the effort that is productive for them.

KEY POINT

It is important that you choose the amount of weight that causes you to fatigue between 6 and 20 reps. As you get stronger, the number of reps doesn't change, but the amount of resistance does!

Number of Sets

A set is a bunch of reps (e.g., 6 to 20). Every group of reps (for example, 6 to 12, 12 to 15, or 15 to 20) to fatigue represents a set. Don't go for conventional wisdom, which says you *have* to do two or three sets, unless you've been doing strength training for a while, are looking for more results, and are willing to invest more time.

Studies have shown that there is little difference between training with one, two, or three sets if you're untrained. (Newer research indicates that even those who are seasoned veterans may experience this same effect.) Any additional increase in muscle gain or strength is minimal for each set performed after the first. Untrained participants will see 80 percent of the gains they'll ever get by doing *one* set of exercise to fatigue for each exercise they perform. Would you get more results if you did more? Yes, but it's a case of diminishing returns.

Eventually (after about three to six months), you'll have to commit more time if you want to take the next step in strength fitness. But initially, one set of exercise will get you strong, give you excellent results, and minimize the time you have to spend lifting.

Frequency of Strength Workouts

You need to strength train a minimum of two times per week, with at least a day of rest between strength workouts. That's it if you're just starting a strength program! Again, research confirms that training two times per week (with one set to fatigue, per exercise) will give a deconditioned person 80 percent of the gains they'd see if they were training three times per week. However, after about three to six months of progressive strength training, you'll probably have to work out about three or four times per week to optimize strength gains. It's easy to maintain strength gains with only a couple of workouts per week.

Number of Exercises

At a minimum, choose 8 to 10 exercises that hit all of the major muscle groups in your body. This leads to equal development in all of your opposing muscles. If you do only arm curls (biceps) and chest presses, you may wreck your posture, and because of the muscular imbalance created, look like a "dork." Choose more exercises if you wish, but using only about 10 exercises doesn't take much time and gets the job done.

Workout Length

If you follow my advice of 6 to 20 reps performed to fatigue, one to two sets of exercise for each major muscle group in the body (which can be accomplished if you wisely choose 8 to 10 exercises), and you lift twice a week, only a 20- to 30-minute time investment for each strength workout is required. This is something you can fit in!

More advanced strength training programs are presented in later chapters. I've presented the minimalist approach here because I want you to know that you don't have to do a lot to get fantastic strength results. That's good news for runners, triathletes, or busy moms and dads who would like to strength train but don't think they have time. If you've been hearing that strength training takes too much time and is hard to do, you've been getting the wrong information!

Exercise Order

Generally, it is best to perform exercise for big muscle groups first, followed by smaller ones. For example, work your hips and buttocks before you work smaller muscles such as the front and back of the thighs, calves, and shins. Go for the chest and back before you "fry" your shoulder and arms. This makes sense because if the small muscles can't contribute to a movement, they become the weak link in an exercise using big muscles. If you fatigue your quads (front of the upper thighs) before you squat or lunge, the quads will tire and give out well before your backside does and you won't give your buttocks a good workout.

On the other hand, after you've trained for several months, it's important to train differently even if your approach is counter to the logic just presented. Always training the same way will limit results and can lead to injury and burnout.

When you're doing a total body workout (working all the muscle groups of the body by choosing 8 to 10 key exercises), the muscle group you start with is not important. Most people do a total body workout when they strength train because they don't have the time to perform split routines (emphasize different body parts over several days) over four or five days. You can begin with your lower body, followed by upper body exercise, and then switch to the abs or back. In fact, hip-hopping around to different body parts is a great idea because it keeps you working out while the body part you just hammered gets a chance to recover. This is called active rest and keeps you from wasting time hanging out until you feel ready to lift again.

Rest Between Sets

If you want to finish your workout in 20 to 30 minutes, you can minimize rest by changing from upper body to lower body and then to ab and back work. The order in which you do this is *not* critical—simply switching from one body part to another unrelated part is what's important. Generally, 30 seconds to two minutes is recommended for recovery from an exercise you just completed to fatigue, if your goal is full recovery before you target this area of the body again. If you hopscotch all over the body as you target muscles, you save time. This is important because most of you have a finite amount of time for working out. This method lets you maximize the amount of time actually spent working out.

Time Between Strength Workouts

Usually a day between strength workouts is about right when you're targeting all of the major muscles. Adequate recovery is essential to avoid hurting yourself and to let your body recover. Though you may have enjoyed a challenging workout, your body's asking you for a chance to grow stronger. If you pound it into submission, you'll never realize the fruits of your hard work.

Table 7.2 details everything you need to know about reps, sets, and rest between sets, as well as the strength results you can expect. Use it to clarify your training direction. Note that an intensity of 12 reps or greater equates to less than 70 percent of a 1-repetition maximum (1-RM). While this load is reasonable to create strength gains, it is not so intense that it would put a deconditioned exerciser at risk for injury. Research indicates that a 10-RM lift equates to about 75 percent of a person's maximum lifting capacity for any given lift. A 6- to 10-RM intensity seems necessary to *optimize* muscular strength and hypertrophy gains, but it's important to progress to these higher percentages of a 1-RM in a progressive manner.

Table 7.2 Strength Chart

Resistance	Result	% 1-RM	Number of reps	Number of sets	Rest between sets
Light	Muscular endurance	< 70	12–20	1–3	20–60 seconds
Moderate	Hypertrophy (increased muscle size) and strength	70–85	6–12	1–6	60–120 seconds
Heavy	Maximum strength and power	85–100	1–6	1–6+	2–5 minutes

Note: Generally, assume a heavier load as soon as you are able to complete the required number of reps listed in the Strength Chart.

Increasing Weight

When you can easily complete more than 6 to 12, 12 to 15, or 15 to 20 repetitions (depending on your current rep range), it's time to up the ante. Add enough weight so that you drop back into the rep framework you're working in (either 6 to 12, 12 to 15, or 15 to 20), but don't add so much that you can't complete the minimum number of reps (6, 12, or 15). *Progressively* increasing how hard you work will keep your mind stimulated, body guessing, muscles pumping, and the results coming!

LIFTING TECHNIQUE

The most important focus of early workouts is *not* to create muscle failure (although this can occur and is an important goal), but to *work on correct exercise technique*. The emphasis on good form gives your muscles a chance to adapt progressively to the demands you're placing on them and lets you learn how to perform exercises correctly before you lift heavier weights.

Lift With Control and Full Range of Motion

With regard to lifting speed, never think "fast." Instead, think "control!" You're lifting in control if you could stop the exercise on a dime if asked. If you leave skid marks or roll into the intersection, you're lifting too fast. Another good guide is to spend two to three seconds lifting a weight in a steady controlled motion followed by three to four seconds lowering the weight, with the same degree of smoothness. I'm not too keen on counting seconds, but if I asked you to stop the movement at any point during a given strength exercise, and you could, this would tell me you're lifting at the correct speed.

KEY POINT

If at any point during a strength training exercise you are asked to stop, you should be able to do so immediately. That defines lifting with control.

Controlling a weight slowly through the fullest range of motion you can attain with comfort will yield the best results with the least risk. Controlled and full-range-of-motion lifting will help you avoid injuring your joints and muscles and maintain flexibility.

Breathe Correctly

First and foremost, breathe regularly during strength training. If you want to get fancy, try to coordinate breathing out when you begin a strength exercise. For example, let's say you're doing a chest press. You're on your back holding a pair of dumbbells. Your goal is to push your arms away from your chest. As you begin to push your arms away, it is natural to hold your breath for a moment. Instead, try to let your breath escape just after, or as you begin, the press. You'll know you're not breathing when you feel the pressure behind your eyeballs start to build, and you begin to wonder when they will explode from your head! If in doubt, breathe, breathe, breathe! Breathe in as you return the weight to your chest.

> ### KEY POINT
>
> Don't think you only get one breath out and one in. Common sense should tell you that it's OK to take small sipping breaths more often if you're lifting with control, which can result in a repetition that takes five or six seconds to complete. Lifting in control requires you to work hard on both phases of your lift.

Holding your breath can cause your blood pressure to rise higher than it should and put unnecessary stress on your heart. You don't need that! Breathing correctly can help you avoid nausea (a polite term that means you feel like dying), dizziness, and the possibility of fainting. At a minimum, just remember to breathe regularly throughout each repetition.

BROOKS'S TOP 15 STRENGTH EXERCISES (AND HOW TO DO THEM)

Not only do these top strength exercises provide you with a strength workout that targets all of the major muscle groups in the body, but you can be confident that you'll be doing them right. In addition, only minimal equipment is needed.

These exercises are sequenced so that you can move from one exercise to the next. Since the same body part is never exercised consecutively, you actively recover while doing the next exercise. More advanced routines sequence exercises differently, but this provides a solid total-body workout.

Supine Dumbbell Press

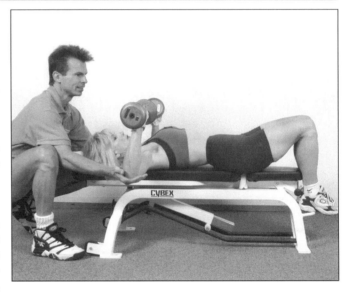

Body Parts Targeted:
Chest, front of the shoulders, back of the arms

Muscles Strengthened:
Pectoralis major, anterior deltoids, triceps

Goals:
To increase strength in the chest and avoid shoulder stress

Setup and Alignment:
Sit upright at one end of a bench, a dumbbell in each hand, with the dumbbells resting on end and in contact with your upper thigh. From this sitting position roll back to a supine (on your back) position and simultaneously cradle the weights to the sides of your chest. Your hands, wrists, and elbows should be close to your sides.

Keep your feet on the floor or on the end of the bench. Your head, shoulder blades, and buttocks should be in firm contact with the bench. Maintain the natural arches in your neck and low back. Pull your shoulder blades toward one another and keep this retracted position throughout your set of repetitions (see photo).

Performing the Exercise:
Press the weights directly above your shoulders. Rotate your shoulders so that your thumbs face one another and your elbows have moved away from your sides. Keep your wrists straight and don't let your dumbbells tilt up or down.

Now, press the weight up as though you're pressing around a fat barrel. Lower the weight until your upper arms are parallel to the ground. Don't let your shoulders rotate forward or back. Then, contract your chest and pull the arms up and back together, while also straightening the elbow. Keep the shoulder blades pulled together and the elbows slightly bent (at the top of the movement) as you finish each repetition.

On your last repetition, move your elbows forward by rotating at the shoulder (the arms are straight) and cradle the weight back to safe position.

Variation:
- From a seated or standing position, attach elastic resistance (tubing) behind you at shoulder height. Although body position has changed, technique does not.

Comments:
A bench that is too high can force you into an extreme arched-back position if you place your feet on the ground. If you need to, place your feet on the bench itself.

Safety Considerations:
Don't lower your upper arms any deeper than parallel to the floor, and keep your elbows from moving in or out. Avoid rounding your upper back by keeping your shoulder blades pulled together. Keep a natural arch in your low back. Keep the setup and alignment throughout the movement.

Kneeling High-Elbow, One-Arm Row

Body Parts Targeted:
Sides of the upper back, back of the shoulder, front of upper arm

Muscles Strengthened:
Latissimus dorsi, posterior deltoid, biceps

Goals:
To strengthen the upper back and back of the shoulder, create muscle balance between the chest and upper back/back of shoulder, and improve posture

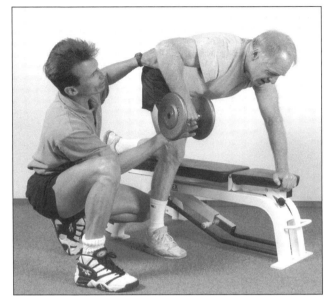

Setup and Alignment:
Place one knee on a bench with the same-side hip aligned directly over it. The knee of the other leg should be at about the same height and slightly bent. Take the hand on the side of the knee that's on the bench and place it just off the edge of the bench, rather than flat on the bench. Your upper body is parallel to the floor.

Lower your body to pick up the weight and return to this start position. Hold the dumbbell without tilting it and keep your wrist straight. Rotate your shoulder so that your elbow is pointing away from your side. Your arms hang straight down and your elbow is slightly bent. Pull your shoulder blades toward one another and keep this retraction throughout the exercise.

Performing the Exercise:
Bend the elbow and pull the arm up until the upper arm is parallel to the floor or higher and the elbow forms a right angle. Pause and slowly return the weight to the floor. Keep the scapulae retracted and elbow pointed away from your side. Return to the starting position. After you've completed your set, repeat on the other side.

Variations:

- The low row with dumbbells emphasizes the latissimus muscle. The starting position is the same except that the dumbbell hangs straight down and the elbow is close to the side. The arm scrapes by the ribs until the upper arm is parallel to the ground or higher.

- The high-elbow row can be performed from a standing or seated position using tubing that is securely attached at shoulder height in front of you.

Safety Considerations:
Don't use momentum. Control the movement and keep your chest square to the floor (the tendency is to open the chest toward the ceiling). Maintain normal curves in your neck and low back. Avoid lifting your head by keeping your head level. Don't rotate your shoulder forward or back (this will change the intended effect of the exercise). Keep the setup and alignment throughout the movement.

Standing Squat

Body Parts Targeted:
Buttocks, front and back of thighs

Muscles Strengthened:
Gluteus maximus, quadriceps, hamstrings

Goals:
To strengthen the buttocks and thighs, improve balance, and increase spinal and upper body stabilizing strength

Setup and Alignment:
Stand upright with your weight over both feet. Your feet should be slightly wider than hip width. Hold a dumbbell in each hand and let your arms hang naturally, straight down and slightly forward of your hips. Starting position calls for your hips and knees to be slightly bent, your trunk to be positioned with a slight forward lean, your head to be neutral, your low back to maintain its normal curve, your shoulder blades to be pulled toward one another, and your weight to be centered over your ankles.

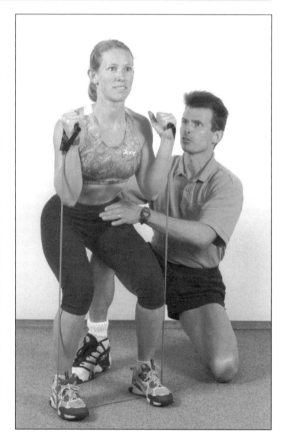

Performing the Exercise:
Bend your knees and slowly move your hips back. Maintain the natural curve in your low back and the slight forward lean of your upper body. Don't round your low back, but lean from the hip. Keep your chest lifted by squeezing your shoulder blades toward one another. The knees should not travel beyond the toes and should follow the direction the toes are pointing. A return to the upright starting position requires control.

Variations:
- Dumbbells may be held at the shoulders, or one dumbbell can be held in front of the body with the arms straight and hanging close to the body and the elbows slightly bent. Technique remains the same.
- Tubing can be used by grasping its handles and placing the cord securely under your feet. Technique stays the same but I recommend that you load and unload (release) the tubing at shoulder height in the lowered position. This will reduce the tension on the tubing and make it easier to get in and out of position.

Safety Considerations:
Keep your back neutral (slightly arched) and your heels on the ground. Align your knees in the direction your feet are pointed and keep the knees aligned over your feet. Go no deeper than 90 degrees or the point at which your upper thighs are parallel to the floor. Keep the setup and alignment throughout the movement. Don't consider placing blocks or weight plates under your heels. This places unnecessary stress on the knees. Maintain the natural arch in your low back. If the back rounds and the hips roll under, go no lower because this is very stressful to the low back.

strength exercise
4

Seated Press Overhead

Body Parts Targeted:
Front of the shoulders, back of the upper arm, upper neck area

Muscles Strengthened:
Anterior deltoid, triceps, upper trapezius

Goals:
To strengthen the front of the shoulders and chest (to a limited extent)

Setup and Alignment:
Set your incline bench at 20 to 30 degrees of incline. Sit with a dumbbell in each hand. The dumbbells rest on end and are in contact with your upper thighs. In this position of inclined support, place your head, shoulder blades, and buttocks firmly against the bench and maintain the natural curves of the neck and low back. Raise the dumbbells to shoulder height and split the difference between having your elbows extremely open and your elbows close to your sides.

Performing the Exercise:
Initiate the press overhead from the starting position. Keep the weights from tilting and perpendicular to the floor. Press the weight up as if you're pressing around a fat barrel. Finish the press by bringing the thumbs toward each other. The dumbbells may or may not touch. Lower with control to the starting position and repeat.

Variation:

• From a seated position on a bench or inclined step, wrap tubing from under the bench seat or step platform top so that it is secure and you have an end in each hand. Sit upright and press slightly up and forward.

Comments:
The angle of the bench, dictates the amount of involvement of the pectoralis major muscle (chest). As the incline is lowered toward horizontal, the "pec major" will become increasingly involved.

Safety Considerations:
Do not set the bench directly vertical (straight up). Pressing directly overhead or behind the neck can put unnecessary stress on the shoulder joint, and do not work the front of the shoulder more effectively.

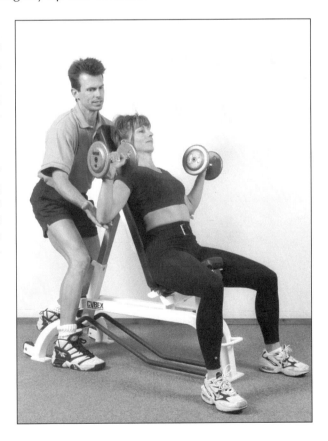

strength exercise 5

Sidelying Lateral Abdominal Curl

Body Parts Targeted:
Abdominals, low back

Muscles Strengthened:
Obliques, rectus abdominis, quadratus lumborum, erector spinae

Goals:
To strengthen the lateral (outside) fibers of the obliques and to create balanced strength between the rectus abdominis and the obliques, to create stabilizing abdominal strength, and to strengthen the low back

Setup and Alignment:
Lie on your side and place a rolled-up towel under your waist (this allows more movement to occur). Place your hands behind your head, with the side of your head resting on the arm that is in contact with the floor. Move your top leg slightly forward and press the foot of the top leg firmly against the floor for stability. The bottom leg is straight or slightly bent. Your shoulders should be aligned with your hips (don't bend at the waist or hips!).

Performing the Exercise:
From this sidelying position, concentrate on drawing the bottom of your rib cage toward the top of the hip. Without letting your hips move forward or backward, lift only as high as the muscles will take you. Return with control to the starting position.

Comments:
This movement is very small and precise. Don't be tempted to use poor or unsafe technique to create lots of motion. These muscles are used more as functional stabilizers (they keep your pelvis and back properly positioned), so remember to let the muscles on the front and back of your trunk— and nothing else!—move you. Don't let your top hip roll forward or back. This takes the emphasis away from the obliques and back muscles. Keep your top elbow and hip oriented to the ceiling.

Safety Considerations:
Don't tilt your head toward the ceiling. Your ears should stay level with your shoulders and go along for the ride as your trunk muscles pull your rib cage toward the hip and raise the upper body slightly off the ground. Keep the setup and alignment throughout the movement.

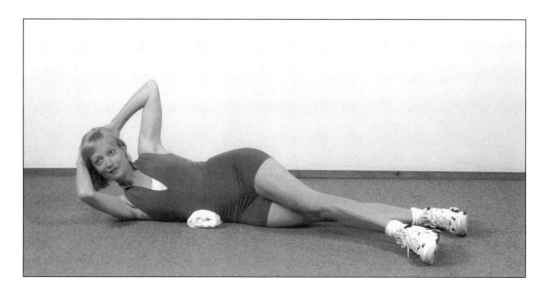

Standing Biceps Curl

Body Part Targeted:
Front of the upper arm (elbow flexors)

Muscles Strengthened:
Elbow flexors group (primarily biceps brachii)

Goal:
To strengthen the front of the upper arm, in isolation

Setup and Alignment:
Stand in an upright position with your feet about shoulder-width apart and knees slightly flexed (keep your head and shoulders over your hips, not forward of them). Let your arms hang naturally to your sides. Palms forward, the upper arms close to your sides (lightly touching), and the lower arms angled away from the body and are wider than the hips. This places your shoulder in a comfortable position and maintains the true hinge-joint action of the elbows. Pull your shoulder blades toward one another. Keep the same shoulder and wrist position throughout the exercise.

Performing the Exercise:
Begin with the elbows slightly bent and wrists straight. Contract the biceps and bring your hands toward your shoulders. Do not lean back and push the hips forward. Instead, maintain tension in your abs and keep your head, shoulders, and hips over your feet (this will keep the work focused in the biceps and not put your low back at risk). Return and repeat.

Variations:

- Dumbbells or tubing allow you to use two other grips— the hammer or neutral grip (thumbs facing forward) and the overgrip (palms facing down)— to emphasize the degree of muscular involvement by various elbow flexors. Follow the same technique described earlier for either of these hand-position variations. These hand-position variations—under, over, and neutral— simply allow you to activate each of the elbow flexor muscles to a lesser or greater degree.

Safety Considerations:
Stay upright and don't bend at your waist. Keep the setup and alignment throughout the movement.

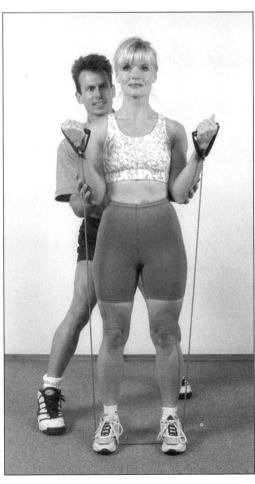

strength exercise 7

Seated Leg Extension

Body Part Targeted:
Front of thigh

Muscles Strengthened:
Quadriceps group (rectus femoris, vastus medialis, vastus intermedius, vastus lateralis)

Goals:
To increase muscular strength in the thigh, to maintain or improve knee joint stability, and to maintain kneecap tracking (correct alignment)

Setup and Alignment:
Adjust the seat so the knees are aligned with the machine's axis of rotation. The leg pad should contact the shin just above the ankle. Sit upright or slightly back with your buttocks pressed firmly against the back pad. Maintain a natural curve in your low back and neck. Squeeze your shoulder blades toward one another and position the legs with a maximum bend of 90 degrees (see illustration). Position your knees in line with your hips and keep your kneecaps oriented to the ceiling (don't let them turn in or out by rotating your hip).

Performing the Exercise:
Relax your ankles and begin to slowly extend the lower legs. Continue straightening the legs until they are fully extended (if your hamstrings are tight, you may not reach full extension). (It is less stressful to the knee to stop about 10 degrees shy of a fully straight leg.) Avoid rotating your hips in or out as this will cause your kneecaps to rotate inward or outward. Return the legs slowly to their starting positions.

Variation:
From a seated position on a bench or inclined step, attach a circular piece of tubing around both ankles. Sit upright and perform the exercise as described.

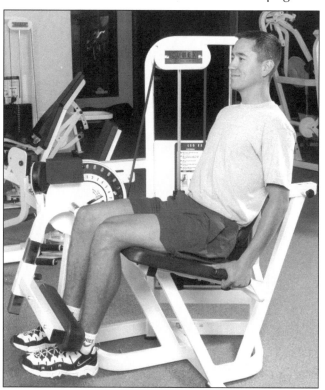

Safety Considerations:
Because this exercise can place considerable stress on the knee joint, it is important to follow the instruction/modifications. Avoid lateral stresses by keeping the kneecaps oriented to the ceiling. This joint motion is also used in the squat, so if you experience knee discomfort or pain, you may want to omit this exercise. Avoid leg extension machines that require you to straighten your knee from a starting position that is greater than 90 degrees (right angle) of knee flexion in relation to the upper leg. Keep the setup and alignment throughout the movement.

strength exercise 8

Prone Spinal Extension

Body Part Targeted:
Low back

Muscle Strengthened:
Erector Spinae

Goals:
To strengthen the low back muscles and increase the structural integrity of the spine

Setup and Alignment:
Position yourself face down with your legs straight and hip-width apart. Rest your forehead on your hands, pointing your elbows to the sides. Pull your shoulder blades together .

Performing the Exercise:
Smoothly lift your upper body off the floor. Keep your shoulder blades pulled together and pulling down toward your buttocks. Lift as high as you can in comfort and without adding momentum (see illustration). Return slowly to the start position.

Variation:

• Perform the same exercise and add rotation. Lift the upper body off the floor slightly before you rotate.

Comments:
Improper spinal alignment can result from weak back muscles and poor posture. This exercise can help counter the effects of sitting with a rounded back.

Safety Considerations:
Keep your hips pressing firmly into the floor and your feet in contact with the floor at all times. Avoid excessive hyperextension of the low back by lifting the upper body off the floor with control. Maintain proper head and neck alignment by keeping your head in contact with your hands. Keep the setup and alignment throughout the movement.

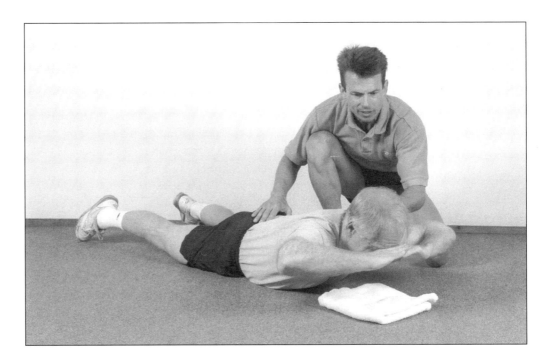

Prone Leg Curl

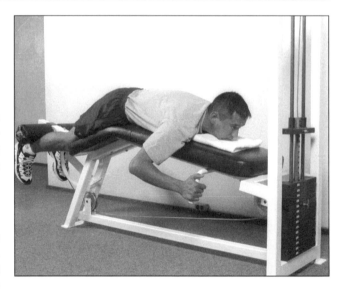

Body Part Targeted:
Back of the upper leg

Muscle Strengthened:
Hamstrings

Goals:
To isolate and strengthen the hamstrings, balance quadriceps strength, stabilize the knee, and help prevent knee injury

Setup and Alignment:
Lie face down on a leg curl machine with your kneecaps just off the edge of the bench. Line both knees up with the rotational axis of the machine. Adjust the roller pads so they contact the back of the legs just above the heel. Keep your kneecaps facing the floor and your knees in line with your buttocks muscles.

Grip the handles lightly, but securely, and press your body firmly against the pad. Your head should face down. (If it is more comfortable to move your head to one side, make sure you switch sides at least once during the set.) Stay with this setup until the exercise ends.

Performing the Exercise:
Begin the exercise with the knees slightly bent and a light contraction in the abdominal muscles. Relax your ankles (neither point your toes nor pull your toes toward your shins). Draw your heels toward your buttocks by contracting the hamstrings and lifting the lower legs up slowly. The heels may or may not touch your buttocks. Return to the starting, slightly bent-knee position.

Variation:

• Lie face down on a comfortable surface with elastic resistance placed around your ankles (flat bands work better than tubing, which has a tendency to roll up your leg). Assume the same setup position. Keep one foot in contact with the ground and draw the other foot toward your buttocks. Return with control and repeat. After completing the desired number of reps, switch to the other leg.

Comments:
As with the quads (seated leg extension), it's best to work the hamstrings unilaterally (one at a time) and bilaterally (both legs at the same time) to promote muscle balance. The tubing variation is a good example of a unilateral leg curl.

Safety Considerations:
Maintain a natural arch in your low back. You don't want to round or excessively arch it. Lift with control and the right amount of weight! This will keep your buttocks from flying and your low back from arching. Start and finish the leg curl with your knees slightly bent. Keep the setup and alignment throughout the movement.

Reverse Abdominal Curl

Body Part Targeted:
Emphasis in the lower region of the abdominals (rectus abdominis)

Muscle Strengthened:
Rectus abdominis, external obliques

Goal:
To control excessive back arch by strengthening the lower region of the rectus abdominis (strong abs can help create good spinal alignment and pelvic stabilization)

Setup and Alignment:
Lie on your back on a comfortable surface and start with your knees bent and over your hips, and a slight curve in your low back. Place your hands alongside you to help provide some balance (don't help by pushing with your arms) and squeeze your shoulder blades together. Do not draw the knees into your chest as you contract your abdominals.

Performing the Exercise:
This small movement is isolated when you contract the abdominals and pull the top of the hips up toward the rib cage. Contract the abdominals enough to flatten the low back and press it firmly into the floor. Continue to pull the pelvis up toward the rib cage, without momentum, until the abs are fully contracted (as far as you can go). Lower with control to the starting position (be sure to release to the natural arch in your low back) and repeat.

Variation:
  • Perform the reverse curl with your head at the high end of an inclined bench. Simultaneously perform a basic curl (crunch) with this reverse ab curl.

Comments:
Technically speaking, there is not an upper and lower abdominal muscle, but the type of ab work you choose can emphasize the upper or lower regions of this one, long muscle called the rectus abdominis. The goal of abdominal work should be to strengthen both the upper and lower regions to help you attain or maintain good spinal alignment.

Safety Considerations:
Keep your knees over your hips and avoid swinging your legs. Perform this small range of motion with absolute control. After each reverse ab curl, return your spine to neutral. Keep the setup and alignment throughout the movement.

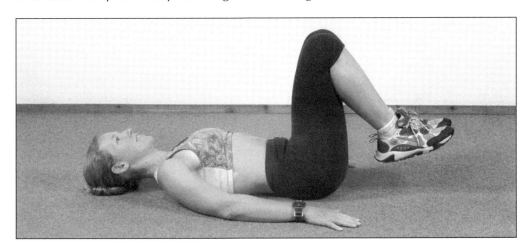

Standing Lateral Raise

Body Part Targeted:
Shoulder

Muscle Strengthened:
Middle deltoid

Goal:
To strengthen the shoulder with middle deltoid emphasis and promote muscular balance in the shoulder.

Setup and Alignment:
From a standing position with your knees and hips slightly bent, weights in hand, place your feet about shoulder-width apart. Your elbows should point back and your weights should not tilt up or down. Let your arms hang naturally to your sides, hands slightly forward of your hips, elbows slightly bent, and lean forward slightly. Maintain the natural curves in your neck and low back and pull your shoulder blades toward one another.

Performing the Exercise:
Maintain a slight elbow bend and move the elbows out to the sides of your body with control. Keep your wrists straight and raise your arms until they are about parallel to the floor. Don't let your shoulders rotate in or out (your elbows will point to the ceiling or floor if you do). Lower and repeat.

Variations:

- Using the same setup, perform the exercise with only one hand lifting weight. Place the opposite hand on your thigh.

- From a standing position, place tubing securely under your feet and grasp each end (or the handles). Perform the exercise as described.

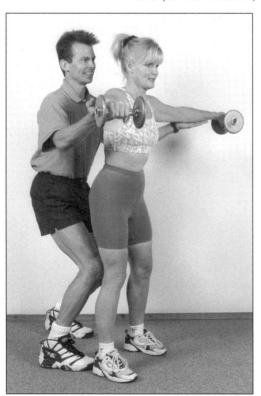

Comments:
Generally, this exercise is performed in an upright position, which more effectively targets the front of the shoulder. This slight technique variation (the lean forward) places the middle deltoid in perfect alignment against the force of gravity and the resistance being placed against it.

Safety Considerations:
Do not round your low back. Raise your upper arms no higher than parallel to the floor. Going no higher can help you avoid a painful situation called shoulder impingement. Keep your thumb from rotating toward the ceiling or floor (avoids any rotation at wrist or shoulder). Keep the setup and alignment throughout the movement.

strength exercise

12

Prone Reverse Hip Lift

Body Part Targeted:
Low back

Muscle Strengthened:
Erector spinae

Goals:
To strengthen the low back muscles and increase the structural integrity of the spine

Setup and Alignment:
Lie face down on a step or platform that is four to eight inches off the floor. The edge of the step should be at or slightly above your waist. Rest your knees on the floor and bend them so that your heels are directly above your knees. Wrap your arms around the sides and top edge of the platform and rest your chin on it. Squeeze your shoulder blades toward one another.

Performing the Exercise:
Keep your waist and chin in contact with the platform and tilt your pelvis forward. (Pad the platform to avoid discomfort when the front of your hips rotate forward.) This action will cause your low back to arch. Lift your knees off the floor as far as you can, with control. Use your low back, not your glutes.

Variation:
- Lie face down on a padded bench/platform that is about 12 inches or more off the floor. This will make the exercise more difficult by increasing available range of motion. Perform the exercise as described.

Comments:
If you have difficulty performing this exercise, position yourself on your hands and knees and practice rounding and arching your back. The arching movement is the feel you want to copy for this exercise.

Safety Considerations:
Use no momentum. Control your movements. Do not simultaneously lift your head and arch your low back. Keep the setup and alignment throughout the movement.

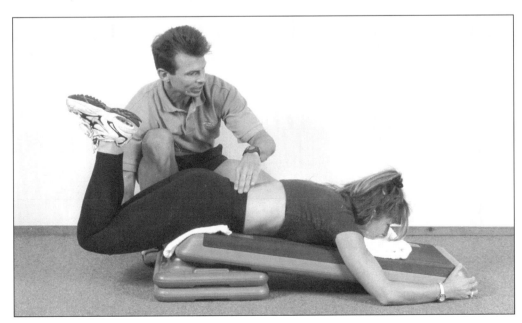

strength exercise 13

Standing Unilateral Heel Raise

Body Part Targeted:
Back of the lower leg

Muscles Strengthened:
Gastrocnemius, soleus

Goal:
To strengthen the lower leg to help prevent injury and improve the functional abilities of these muscles to assist with running, walking, jumping, pushing off, etc., to achieve balance and ankle stability

Setup and Alignment:
Stand next to a platform or step that is about eight inches off the ground. Place the foot closest to the platform on it, for balance only. Your other foot is close to the platform and pointed forward. Keep your head, shoulders, and hips level, and all of your weight over your outside foot (straight leg). Pull your shoulder blades toward one another and keep the natural curves in your neck and low back.

Performing the Exercise:
Keep all of your weight on your straight leg and press your forefoot of the weight-bearing leg into the floor, lifting your heel. All of your body weight should move up, so don't move your hips forward or back, and keep your weight evenly distributed across all five toes. After finishing your set, repeat on the other side.

Variation:
• Hold dumbbells in either hand and perform the same exercise. The dumbbells provide progressive overload so you can continue to get stronger.

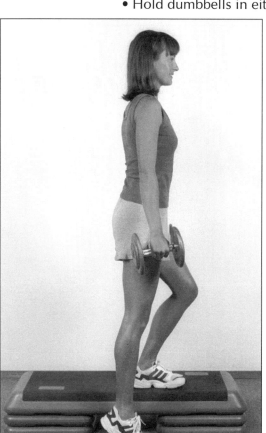

Comments:
Balance the unilateral heel raise with an exercise that targets the front of the lower leg. For example, from a seated position, have your workout partner manually resist your foot as you pull your toe toward your shin. If you don't have a workout partner, attach an ankle weight around the front of your foot.

Safety Considerations:
Keep your toes pointed forward during the heel raise. Turning your toes in or out can stress the ankle and has no advantage with regard to working the lower leg muscles more effectively or differently. Maintain the setup and alignment throughout the movement.

Supine Unilateral Triceps Press

Body Part Targeted:
Back of the upper arm

Muscle Strengthened:
Triceps

Goal:
To strengthen the back of the upper arm, in isolation

Setup and Alignment:
Lie on your back on a bench. Keep your feet on the floor or bring them onto the end of the bench. Maintain the normal curves in your low back and neck. Your head, shoulder blades, and buttocks should be in firm contact with the bench. Pull your shoulder blades toward one another. With weight in one hand, position this arm with the elbow oriented toward the ceiling and keep it there during the entire set. It should not move forward, back, in, or out. Orient your little finger toward the ceiling. Support the raised arm, just above the elbow, with the other hand.

Performing the Exercise:
Perform the exercise with one arm (weight in hand) and support the elbow and shoulder position with the other, as described earlier. Bend the elbow of the working arm by lowering the hand to the side of the head and toward the bench. Press the weight upward (little finger leading) until the arm is fully straightened. Keep your wrists straight and don't let the weight tilt up or down. Return with control and, after completing the set, repeat on the other side.

Comments:
It's easier to perform this exercise using one weight, when compared to performing a bilateral (both arms simultaneously) movement.

Safety Considerations:
Don't let your elbow flare out by keeping your elbow oriented to the ceiling. Lower the weight carefully toward the side of the head and bench. Keep the setup and alignment throughout the movement.

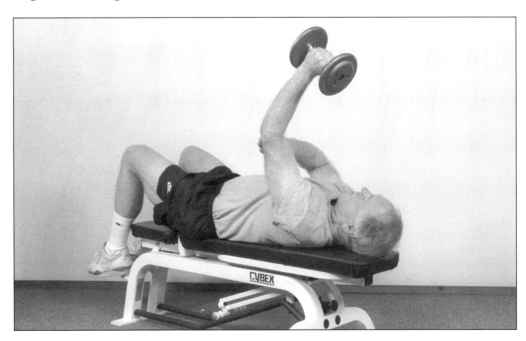

strength exercise 15

Sidelying Rotator Cuff Series (three key exercises from one position)

Body Part Targeted:
Shoulder joint

Muscles Strengthened:
- Supraspinatus (abduction)
- Infraspinatus, teres minor (external rotation)
- subscapularis (internal rotation)

Goal:
To develop shoulder joint strength and structural integrity

Setup and Alignment:

- Lie on your side with a rolled-up towel under your head (1). With the weight in hand, rest your top arm on the side of the body. Place your lower arm in a comfortable position. Maintain a slight bend in the knees and hips and keep the natural curve in your low back.

- After setting up the same way as setup #1, move the top hand so that the arm is bent 90 degrees and the elbow is pressed into the body (2). The elbow stays glued to this spot throughout the exercise.

- From setup position #1 or #2, move the weight from the top hand to the bottom hand (3). Rest the top hand to a resting position on the side of the body. Lower the bottom hand so that the elbow is bent at 90 degrees and the hand is just above the floor. Your bottom elbow stays in contact with the floor throughout the exercise.

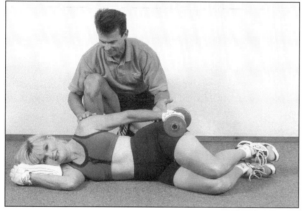

Performing the Exercise:

- From setup #1, keep the wrist and top arm straight. Lift the arm about 45 to 60 degrees directly toward the ceiling and away from your side. Don't let your body roll forward or back. Keep the top arm aligned over the side of your body throughout the exercise. Return the weight with control.

- From setup #2, keep the top arm bent at 90

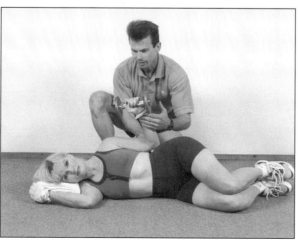

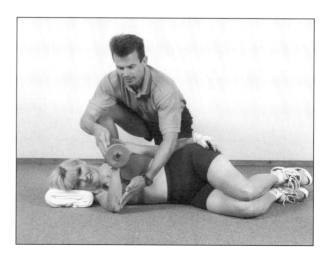

degrees and the elbow in contact with your side. Keep your wrist straight and lower the weight as far as you can without the elbow lifting from your side. Don't let your body roll forward or back. Return the weight with control.

- From setup #3, keep the bottom arm bent at 90 degrees and your elbow in line with your shoulder. Your hand is just off the floor. Rotate your lower arm inwardly.

Comments:
Sufficient rotator cuff muscle strength is the foundation for any upper body strength program or sporting activity that requires the use of the arms, chest, and upper back.

Safety Considerations:

- (1) Support your head so that it is not tilted to either side and maintain the natural curve in your low back. Avoid lying directly on your bottom shoulder by cheating it slightly forward during setup and alignment.

- (2) Keep the upper elbow in its starting position throughout the exercise and pressed into your side (setup #2). Don't rotate your top arm any higher than 90 degrees (top hand oriented to ceiling).

- (3) Keep the lower elbow in its starting position throughout the exercise.

Quick Index:

8 Cross-Train for Variety (and Results!)

Cross-training requires you to use a variety of activities to achieve total body fitness. Total body fitness may not be realized if you use only one type of activity. By using cross-training activities, you can achieve balance in your program, improve your overall fitness level, decrease your risk of injury by avoiding the same workout every day, and maintain enthusiasm for your workouts.

There is no one, best cross-training activity. And that's the beauty! No single exercise can offer all the benefits of a strengthened heart, bones, muscles, and joints; a decreased risk for heart disease; increased muscle and strength; decreased body fat; weight control; and flexibility. Each combination of cross-training exercises offers a unique set of training benefits for your mind and body.

The term *cross-training* has been around for a long time, but this concept of varying your workout choices and activities still commands serious consideration. Whether you are a professional or recreational athlete, you should cross-train to avoid overuse injury, keep yourself interested and excited about your training, and provide different physical stimulation that will keep the results coming. Cross-training should provide you with the right amount of variety and challenge that will keep you checking off your fitness goals in a safe and fulfilling way.

Cross-training, like periodization, is planned and results oriented. Cross-training emphasizes variety and balance with regard to activity choices. Periodization focuses on changing how often, how long, and how hard you work out over specific time periods while including planned days of rest and recovery. Cross-training can be a valuable part of a periodization program.

KEY POINT

Plan cross-training into your program. Don't wait until you think you need a change of pace.

TYPES OF CROSS-TRAINING

Even if a favorite activity is the foundation of your program, a well-rounded and balanced approach requires you not only to cross-train between the major components of fitness (cardio, strength, flexibility), but also to switch the activities within each of these components. Plan changes into your program in addition to adding them to your workout when the mood grabs you! A switch in the program can be formally planned into your long-term program or spontaneous. For example, rather than taking your usual walk, add a combination of walking and running, or change from a barbell or machine chest press to a dumbbell press, just because you feel like it. Also, periodize (formally plan) your program to include, for example, outdoor training if a majority of your training occurs indoors. You get the idea! While still accomplishing your workout goals, you've added the key element of variety. Whether formal or spontaneous, cross-training brings in newness and fresh energy. It will stimulate both your mind and your body.

Cross-Training Between Components of Fitness

A program consisting exclusively of running will give you a high level of cardiovascular fitness but will increase your risk of injury and mental burnout. It does not address the important fitness components of strength and flexibility. If you only strength train, you're missing the important contributions regular cardiovascular training can give you, for example, reducing your chances of having a heart attack and helping you with weight loss. In addition, you're missing out on the great benefits stretching brings to your program.

By cross-training with a variety of activities between all of the major components of fitness, you can improve your cardiovascular fitness, muscle strength and endurance, and flexibility; decrease your body fat; and increase your muscle mass, all in a time-efficient manner. Cross-training leads to a well-rounded development of your body and balanced fitness.

Cross-Training Within Components of Fitness

Even if you're cross-training between the key components of balanced fitness, that's not quite enough. You also need to change activity and exercises within each area of fitness. If you always bike, do the same 10 strength exercises on machines, and perform the same five stretches after every workout, you could argue that you're cross-training. Yes, you are training between the three major areas of fitness, but you need to broaden your approach. Doing the same old workout day in and day out will put you on the road to injury, lack of results, and mental burnout!

KEY POINT

If you start to view your workouts as a prison sentence rather than approaching them with unbridled enthusiasm, it's time to introduce cross-training into your program planning process.

To cross-train among the major components of fitness, you need to find several cardio activities you like (aerobic cross-training); use machines, weights, tubing, and different exercises in your strength training (strength cross-training); and stretch in a variety of ways and places (i.e., outdoors versus indoors and standing versus lying down). Even though stretching (or for that matter, exercising in general) inside or outside is not really that different, a change of scenery can give you a big mental boost and lift you out of the "routine rut."

With regard to stretching, you may also want to explore yoga and the use of a combination of massage and passive stretching sessions. It's too easy to slack up on a regular stretching program. Use a variety of approaches and methods to keep you on track, interested, seeing results, and excited about all of the areas of fitness that are important parts of a balanced approach to fitness.

GETTING STARTED IN CROSS-TRAINING

As is true for any new exercise, start gradually. Let's say the cornerstone activity of your training is cycling. You may be very fit in a particular activity, but different exercises use different muscles and motions. Doing too much too soon will lead to unnecessary soreness and even injury.

Cross-training has been likened to "fitness grazing." It's fun to create a collection of fitness activities under each area of fitness (cardio, strength, flexibility) that you enjoy and can insert into your programs when change and variation are appropriate. However, cross-training should probably be done in moderation with specific goals for fitness improvement or, possibly more important, recovery. Cross-training can improve your mental outlook and certain aspects of performance if you approach it properly.

I emphasize a conservative starting point. For example, if you're a fit cyclist, don't start a running program at the same levels of intensity and duration! If you're adding strength training to a running program, carefully consider the number of times you train this component of fitness per week and the amount of resistance you'll be using. This seems obvious and prudent, but many people make the mistake of being competitive and overzealous. Use a smart and conservative progression in the new activity. Finally, don't try to be a champion or match your performance to your main sport or activity. Keep your goals sensible and have fun!

USING CROSS-TRAINING

Most people increase the intensity of their workouts by running faster or lifting more weight. However, if you simply need a little variety, try cross-training without initially changing the intensity, or how hard you work. This technique works especially well with strength and stretching programs or cardiovascular circuit training workouts.

An easy first step with a strength training program is to change the sequence of strength exercises that you're already doing to create variety and a new overload (intensity). Even though you haven't introduced any new exercises or increased intensity (more resistance), experts theorize that the fatigue pattern of the involved motor units (groups of muscle fibers within a muscle) changes, causing them to adapt to what the muscles perceive as a new stimulus. It is as though the muscles think they are working differently and responding to a new strength stimulus (and they are!). This translates into results for you!

Another option would be to replace all the exercises, or those you think necessary, in the strength routine with new ones. Take care to replace each exercise with one that targets the same muscle group(s) to preserve balance.

For example, a bench press can be replaced by push-ups, dumbbell presses, incline and decline presses, or dumbbell or elastic resistance chest flyes. Any changes in movement patterns, even if you are targeting the same muscle group(s) and using similar joint actions, will require the muscle to respond differently. This holds true even if you don't change the number of reps you perform to fatigue (i.e., work harder). Simply changing exercises can act as a stimulus (overload) to create further strength gains, without simultaneously increasing resistance.

You might be thinking, what happens with other components of fitness? If you replace one stretch for another that targets the same body area or switch from biking to rowing and keep the intensity of the exercise the same (same tension on the muscles being stretched or similar heart rate/RPE), the principle discussed in the previous paragraph holds true. So, even though it is appropriate to change intensity by going harder, longer, and faster, it isn't the only approach that will give you increases in your body's perception of how hard you are working.

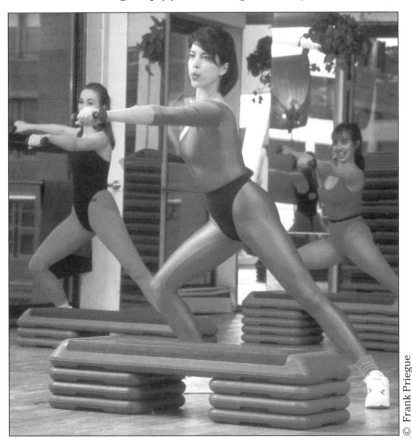

© Frank Priegue

Step aerobics is just one of many exersises you can choose to add variety to your cross-training.

Cross-training *within* the muscular strength and endurance component can positively affect compliance, motivation, and interest, as well as stimulate the body toward additional strength gains. For optimal muscular development, variety is the name of the game.

When cross-training in the cardiovascular component of fitness, any aerobic activity can replace the one you're using. Always start at a lesser intensity, relative to heart rate or your perceived exertion, and don't approach the program with the same vigor with which you attacked your former activity.

Finally, use a variety of stretching/yoga exercises to challenge your mind and body optimally. When changing stretches, follow the same rules (i.e., breathe continually, sustain tolerable tension on the muscle, and hold the stretches for about 10 to 60 seconds without bouncing).

TARGETED CROSS-TRAINING

For many years, cross-training has conflicted with the time-honored, science-based principle of specificity. In other words, if you want training results, align your training activities to closely mimic those of the sport in which you want to improve (for example, to be a good distance runner, run long distances). To further punctuate this belief, many physiologists believed that other cardiovascular activities or strength training would largely be a waste of time if your goal was to "run long." However, many physiologists (including myself) now believe (with good science to back us) that cross-training can help you attain optimal performance and fitness results.

Optimal training in any activity results from a combination of many physical attributes. Optimal physical performance requires some combination of cardiovascular (aerobic and anaerobic), strength, and flexibility fitness. Even a long-distance marathon runner needs anaerobic cardiovascular conditioning to sprint at the finish line or to strategically move herself up in a pack of runners. In addition, upper body, abdominal, and back strength training will assist her in maintaining good posture. Upper body muscle fatigue leads to loss of form and slower running speeds. Flexibility is essential in the lower legs, hips, and thighs to prevent injury and to encourage proper body position and stride length.

If your goal is to excel in a single sport endeavor, a majority of your training should be spent training in that sport or activity. But within a periodized program, cross-training still plays an important role in at least maintaining your fitness level, decreasing the risk of overuse injury that could result from doing the same repetitive actions on a daily basis, and providing fun and varied recovery activity.

SAMPLE CROSS-TRAINING PLAN

How you use cross-training will vary depending on your goals and fitness activity interests. The point is to use it to some degree in your program. This is true regardless of whether your goals are performance or health/fitness oriented. You need to find several activities you like, ones that target all of the

Table 8.1 Sample Cross-Training Plan

Day	Workout Activities	Time/Distance
Monday	Warm-up, light stretch, 10K run (moderate, 7.5-minute pace), cool-down, stretch	45 minutes/6 miles
Tuesday	Circuit strength training using machines, all major muscle groups, one set, 12–15 reps; stretch and cool-down	25 minutes
Wednesday	Interval workout at the track: 3-mile warm-up and stretching; 90-second anaerobic emphasis; 15-minute running cool-down and stretching	60 minutes
Thursday	Warm-up 20 minutes cycling, slow pace; circuit train using free weights, all major muscle groups with emphasis on abdominals and low back, one set, 12–15 reps; stretch and cool-down	45 minutes
Friday	Swimming, moderate pace; cool-down with stretch on swimming deck	45 minutes
Saturday	Long run at race pace (6-minute mile); cool-down with 20-minute concentrated stretch emphasizing hip flexor, hamstrings, and calf stretches	90 minutes/15 miles
Sunday	Morning hike in the hills with family	4 or 5 hours

important areas of fitness, so that you can attain optimal and well-rounded fitness (see table 8.1 above).

A program without cross-training is like eating bland cereal for breakfast, lunch, and dinner. While you may love your "jump start" breakfast of healthy cereal with nonfat milk and yogurt in the morning, you probably don't want it at every meal. In fact, in time you would probably grow to despise it and dread the drudgery of meal time! The same holds true for your training schedule.

All of us have our favorite activities that create the foundation of our workouts. Runners love to run, walkers and hikers love to walk, bikers love to bike, and swimmers love to swim. Nevertheless, exercise variety will breathe a freshness into your workouts you cannot imagine until you try it. If you're already cross-training, keep it up. If you're resistant to the idea, give it a shot and you'll never go back. Cross-training helps to optimize your training results and keeps you excited about coming back for more!

Quick Index:

9 Build in Rest and Recovery

Don't feel guilty. Rest and recovery is not the same as skipping a workout. Successful athletes on every level build this crucial component into their training programs.

While you already know that you have to progressively challenge your body with activity if you want to build your fitness, here's a surprise: the actual physiological gains occur during rest and recovery!

OK, now I bet you're listening. Rest and recovery are essential elements in your training program and should be carefully accounted for if you want to realize optimal results. Use rest and active recovery along with proper exercise variety and variation and you will take your workout efforts to new heights and produce greater results than you will if you only concentrate on work!

This restorative aspect of your workout program is at least 50 percent of the result equation, if not more. This is often a hard lesson to be learned by a well-intentioned, dedicated exerciser who pushes every workout or daily pounds himself into submission. Remember, recovery does not necessarily mean taking a nap. It represents a balance you need to develop, including working out at varying intensities and using a variety of activities. Recovery will enhance your training results. Incredible as it may seem, doing less in terms of intensity will give you a better return for your workout efforts. Once you learn and experience the magic of recovery combined with the right combination of effort, you'll never go back to your old ways.

REPAIRING AND BUILDING YOUR BODY

Does a negative result in a positive? From a physiological perspective, the answer is no.

For example, it is often said that during strength training you break down the muscle and then it rebuilds stronger. This implies that the stimulus for change or training result is damage (a negative). While some damage to the muscle tissue may be an inevitable result of a tough workout, damage in itself is not the stimulus for change. Instead, the right overload to which the body is not accustomed is the key. Note that high repetition (i.e., about 20-plus repetitions) strength programs that use light weights produce little hypertrophy, but muscle damage (soreness) can still occur from, for example, swinging the weights in an uncontrolled fashion.

It is very important to note that the process of hypertrophy (increased muscle size) is directly related to the *synthesis* (putting together) of cellular material. The word *synthesis* implies that strength training is a positive building process (anabolic), rather than a negative, or catabolic, process.

To further emphasize that training is a positive process, think about the following example. You can overstretch a muscle and create soreness, which is more accurately identified as muscle damage or microtrauma. However, damaging muscle in any training scenario (cardio, strength, or flexibility fitness training) does not represent the proper and specific overload stimulus (i.e., how hard, how long, how often) to cause positive growth and nervous system adaptations. Additionally, the fibers are more susceptible to recurrent injury because of related scarring in muscle tissue that is associated with muscle damage and a resultant decreased blood supply to the scarred area because of accumulated trauma.

> ### KEY POINT
>
> Approach your training with the idea that you should do all you can to avoid extreme soreness or microtrauma while training hard enough to continue producing training results. If you avoid damage, you won't have to stop training to repair! To achieve maximal training results, rest must be carefully planned, monitored, and adhered to within your training plan. Don't blow it off because you feel good.

TYPES OF ACTIVE RECOVERY

Active recovery is productive recuperation from day to day, week to week, month to month, or even between exercises. It is an excellent method for avoiding overtraining and maximizing your time. As we have seen, active recovery is a key component of periodization.

Active recovery, or active rest, is usually performed at lower intensities of effort and duration than are used for regular exercise. You should consider using different activities, at least part of the time, for this recovery and restoration time period.

> **KEY POINT**
>
> Active recovery allows for physical recovery and enhancement of the adaptation process. Effort is 50 percent of the training equation, and recovery and restoration is the other important half!

Another type of active recovery occurs between exercises and within a given training session. Many of your health, fitness, and performance goals can be optimized by using active recovery between sets of strength exercises. This allows for a more productive use of limited time. For example, a stretching exercise or exercising another body part can serve to facilitate recovery from a previous strength exercise without requiring total inactivity.

AVOIDING OVERTRAINING

A basic principle of training is to stress, or overload, the physiological system (your body). Positive overloads cause the body to respond with, for example, increases in strength, muscular endurance, and cardiovascular capacity. Because of this basic training principle—progressive increases in overload—there is a risk of overtraining. It can lead to staleness, exhaustion, and injury.

People who are extremely driven are susceptible to overtraining. Attempting to perform your best during every training session and being motivated to extend this effort regardless of how you feel invites injury or emotional burnout. Nothing will shut down the training process and compliance more quickly than this scenario.

The underlying causes of overtraining or staleness (mental and physical) are a combination of emotional and physical factors. The emotional demands of life, family pressures, a personal desire to excel at every undertaking, and the expectations of significant others can be sources of intolerable emotional stress. In addition to the stress of exercise and training, environmental factors such as heat stress and improper nutrition may also lead to overtraining symptoms.

When planning your program, consider the *total* stress you're under. For example, during tax season an accountant may be more susceptible to overtraining. Much like heart disease, which develops insidiously, overtraining exhibits no preliminary warning symptoms. By the time you realize it, you've pushed too hard and the damage is already done.

While training intensity (e.g., speed of running or amount of weight lifted) is *potentially* more stressful than training volume (reps, more days, duration of each session), excess in either, or simultaneous increases in intensity and volume, may lead to overuse injuries and overtraining.

> **KEY POINT**
>
> Prevention is always preferable to the challenge of attempting to remedy the psychological and physiological state of being overtrained or injured.

An excellent way to minimize the risk of overstressing is to follow cyclic (periodization) training procedures. Periodization alternates easy, moderate, and harder periods of training over specific time frames. As a general rule, one or two days of hard training should be followed by an equal number of easy days.

The importance of variety, cross-training, active recovery, and actual days of rest for the mind and body cannot be overemphasized. The optimal adaptive response (results from your training) often occurs when your training is mixed with new activities and recovery.

IDENTIFYING OVERTRAINING

The most common symptoms of overtraining are feelings of heaviness and the inability to perform well and concentrate. Working out is no longer a joy; it has turned into a struggle. Other warning signs are listed in the box below. If you feel this situation exists, it is time to make some immediate changes in your approach to working out.

Idiosyncratic personality variables and mood swings (you know your own personality) and day-to-day variations in the *sensations* of fatigue should not be confused with overtraining. It is OK for you to feel tired or challenged from a workout. It is not uncommon to feel heavy after a day of hard training. These are often short-lived sensations that dissipate before the next training session. Coupled with rest, a light day or no training after the hard session, and proper nutrition, these symptoms are usually relieved. By keeping track of these general indicators and erring on the side of caution, you can prevent most cases of overtraining.

Overtraining Warning Signs

Health Signs

- Elevated resting heart rate, blood pressure, or both
- Generalized body aches and pain
- Head colds (especially if chronic), allergic reactions, or both
- Body weight loss with decreased appetite
- Occasional nausea

Life Signs

- Personal problems, increased tension, anger, irritability (you're hard to be around!)
- No interest in activities you usually enjoy
- Sleep disturbances (loss of sleep)

Training Signs

- Loss of motivation to train, or staleness
- Cutting sessions short: an hour seems too long!
- Loss of performance
- Unusual muscle soreness and tenderness after training
- Fatigue lingers during workout and throughout the day
- Recovery takes longer immediately after the workout

Using Heart Rate as an Indicator of Overtraining

It is not surprising that overtraining has a dramatic effect on the energy demands for a given submaximal exercise bout. When you are beginning to cross the line of being overtrained, you will find that your heart rate for a given effort is significantly higher. For instance, if your heart rate (HR) for a workload of 5 mph on a treadmill is normally 135 beats per minute (bpm), this same level of effort might increase to 145 bpm. You're not losing your aerobic fitness, but skill, form, and efficiency of movement may be deteriorating. The best and most practical way for you to monitor overtraining is to observe heart rate response during activity or rest.

Heart Rate During Activity as an Indicator of Overtraining

To use heart rate during activity as an indicator of overtraining, follow three steps:

1. Record your heart rate (HR) at a fixed pace and load (resistance) on any piece of cardiovascular equipment at the *onset* of training or *prior* to a new phase in your program. This is called the untrained heart rate response (UT).

2. Record your HR at the same given pace and load and on the same piece of equipment any time *after* significant and progressive training. This is called the trained heart rate response (TR).

3. Record your HR at the same fixed pace and overload and on the same piece of equipment during any period when you demonstrate symptoms of being overtrained. This is called the overtrained heart rate response (OT).

You will usually find the UT heart rate to be highest, followed by the OT and finally the TR heart rate. These results indicate that the TR heart rate was most efficient for the pace and overload on that particular piece of equipment. The OT heart rate was higher than the TR rate because of overtraining, but was still lower or more efficient than the initial untrained state (UT). Based on heart rate response to given workloads, you can objectively monitor the direction of training so that it remains beneficial. This kind of data and observation may provide a warning signal for overtraining. Whenever you record a heart rate that is 5-10 percent higher than your TR heart rate, it's time to evaluate your program. You're at risk for overtraining.

Heart Rate During Rest as an Indicator of Overtraining

Take your pulse while still in bed. Locate your radial pulse (thumb side, near your wrist) and count your heart beats for 60 seconds. If your resting heart rate is 10 percent above normal (your normal resting heart rate should be determined when you're not exhausted, sick, or feeling overtrained), it indicates you may be overtrained. Though you may be feeling fine, it's probably a good idea to pay close attention to nutrition and moderate (think "cruise") your training. If your resting heart rate is 20 percent above normal, take the day off or drastically cut back on your workout (you're probably not feeling top notch, anyway).

Avoiding Overtraining With Sensible Progression

By piling on too much too soon you run the risk of becoming discouraged or injured. Keep the following points in mind when planning your workouts to avoid falling into this trap:

1. Allow about two weeks to get used to any increase in level of effort before making the workout any harder or longer. This is especially true for those just starting to work out.
2. Do not progress to harder workouts if you feel any extreme soreness or stiffness.
3. When increasing amount of weight lifted or duration of cardiovascular efforts, do not increase by more than about 5 percent.
4. Sensible progression cannot occur too slowly. Remember, your commitment to exercise is for a lifetime. Patience is the rule if you want to avoid injury and discomfort during exercise.

RECOVERING FROM OVERTRAINING

Relief from overtraining usually comes from a significant reduction in training intensity, a change of activity, or complete rest. Many coaches and trainers generally suggest a few days of easy training using the same activity. Many experts, to the contrary, observe that participants recover faster when they rest completely or engage in some other form of very low intensity exercise. Try emphasizing stretching and relaxation, or just take the break. It doesn't help to slog through what I call a garbage workout!

> **KEY POINT**
>
> If you suspect overtraining, take a day off from training, introduce variety, or at least cut back in how long and how hard you work out.

Recording how you feel during and after your workout is important when keeping an exercise diary. A quick look back at a previous workout will help you monitor heart rate, weight lifted, and so on, and how you felt. For instance, if your heart rate was 10 beats higher for your usual three-mile run and your legs felt like lead, you could be approaching an overtrained state.

KNOWING WHEN TO QUIT

You will rarely hear me utter this four-letter word, but there is a time and place to quit. Should you become injured, or even think the possibility exists as a result of overtraining, you should contact your doctor. She can help you distinguish between normal postexercise discomfort and pain related to injury. It is important to prevent further injury (stop and seek counsel) and to get you back on track with your exercise program as soon as possible after an injury, but first you must heal.

The following pain levels and practical pointers can help you make the right decision with regard to exercising, contacting your doctor, or just saying no (See the *Penn State Sports Medicine Newsletter*, June 1997.)

Level 1: Pain that is present after you've finished exercising but goes away that same day

Level 2: Pain that starts during exercise but isn't so bad that you can't keep going

Level 3: Pain that starts during exercise but really limits what you can do and eventually keeps you from continuing

Level 4: Pain that continues even when you're not exercising and you're constantly reminded of it with even the slightest physical activity

Without attempting to play doctor (if you have any doubts or concerns, always contact your doctor), levels 1 and 2 can usually be countered with ice application, a reduction in exercise duration and intensity, gentle stretching, and over-the-counter pain killers or analgesics (i.e., ibuprofen found in Advil and Nuprin). It should be noted that ibuprofen effectively fights pain and inflammation. Products containing acetaminophen, such as Tylenol, can reduce or eliminate pain but have no anti-inflammatory action. Often, the key to reducing the effects of initial and further injury is to limit swelling. Ice, elevating the injured body part, and anti-inflammatory medicine can be highly effective.

The key is not to exacerbate the situation by being too aggressive with your workouts or ignoring obvious pain signals. If the pain and discomfort becomes great enough, it is often self-limiting. In other words, if you have any common sense left and are listening to your body, you will take the sensible approach and STOP! If you are experiencing the symptoms associated with pain levels 3 or 4, seek medical advice from a qualified health care professional.

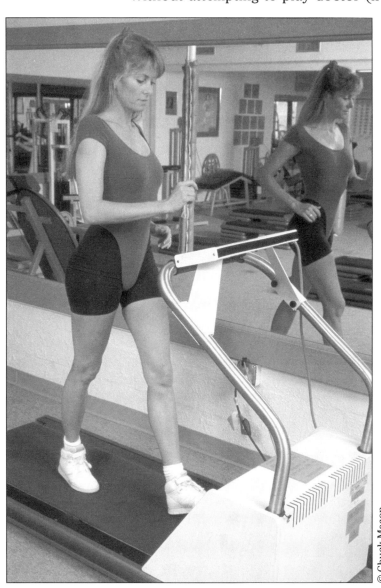

© Chuck Mason

Fatigue may be a sign of overtraining, but don't push yourself through real pain.

LAST WORDS ON OVERTRAINING

Don't let exercise become a negative addiction that keeps you from listening to your body. Know when to pull back. Familiarize yourself—well—with this chapter. If you think you're approaching the brink of overtraining, make the appropriate changes in your workout plans. If have even the slightest suspicion that you may have been injured as a result of your training program (overtraining or otherwise), contact your doctor. Staleness from overtraining can have serious consequences for your physical and mental health.

Overtraining, once known only in the athlete's arena, is being seen more often with well-intentioned, committed exercisers who ignore the obvious warning signs and symptoms. If you're always feeling sluggish, not eating, sleeping poorly, depressed, feeling as if you've got the weight of the world on your shoulders (everything is work and a big effort!), wrung out, worn out, and don't even want to be around yourself, the solution is simple: take some time off!

Quick Index:

10 Fuel Your Workouts

Not getting the performance results you want or the physical changes in your body—such as fat loss and muscle gain—that you think you deserve? Feel a little flat or burned out? If your answer is yes, and you're doing all the right physical things in your workout such as working out at the right level of effort; mixing your activity by cross-training; balancing your workouts by doing cardio, strength, and stretching exercises; and periodizing (allowing for recovery and hard effort) your program—it's time to consider your eating habits.

EATING FOR EXERCISE

Regardless of what you may have heard, eating for exercise is not very different from eating for your personal health and well-being. To be sure, there are a few tricks to fueling yourself before, during, and after exercise, but the foundational part of your diet (which should be low-fat) should not change, whether your goal is to feel better, lose weight, achieve optimal health, or improve your performance.

Too many athletes and recreational exercisers take their regimens to unhealthy and unsafe extremes. There is a smart approach to timing the ingestion and quantity (ratio of carbohydrates, fats, and protein) of nutrients that is based on science and what is known to work with your body's nutritional needs.

If the words *strict* or *religion* come to mind with reference to your dietary approach, replace these words with *consistent* or maybe *disciplined* and use the 80/20 rule. In other words, follow your eating and exercise plan 80 percent of the time, and don't worry if you slip 20 percent of the time.

The 80/20 rule replaces the 90/10 rule I used to follow. That is, 90 percent of the time I used to make healthy choices and 10 percent of the time I didn't. Over the years I have realized that my personal training clients, as well as I, need to bend the 90/10 rule more if an approach to healthier eating is going to work in a real-life, practical sense. With the addition of two young sons, my personal 90/10 rule changed to 80/20 and has even eroded to 70/30 on occasion. It's funny how a family can impact your eating habits. However, you can still eat healthfully and perform at high levels by eating right *most* of the time.

Don't set yourself up for failure by trying to be perfect all of the time. Approaching personal health, exercise, nutrition, eating habits, and food choices with an all-or-none attitude is the perfect setup for personal failure. Eating should not be approached from the fringe of extreme choices. Perfection is *not* normal. Many distractions in the form of travel, job, and family may come up on a daily basis.

KEY POINT

Everyone needs some operating room to enjoy eating and to be successful at making healthy nutritional choices. You need a flexible, nonobsessive approach to nutrition (and for that matter, exercise) that encourages consistency, not perfection.

COMPUTING YOUR CALORIES

Have you always guessed or never even considered the number of calories you should be eating every day? Following are two easy ways to determine your calorie needs.

Estimating Your Daily Calorie Requirement

The following four steps can help you estimate your daily calorie requirement.

1. Determine your resting metabolic rate (RMR) by multiplying your body weight by 10.

$$\text{Current body weight} \times 10 = \text{RMR}$$

RMR represents the number of calories it takes to keep your body humming along all day long. Your body's RMR can total as much as 75 percent of the calories you burn all day simply by maintaining bodily functions such as producing new skin cells, breathing, making new red blood cells, and keeping your heart pumping. If you weighed 155 pounds, this is how it works:

$$155 \times 10 = 1550 = \text{RMR}$$

2. Estimate how many calories you need for your formal, or scheduled and planned, exercise each day.

Estimate your physical activity energy expenditure by using the following calorie assignments. For an activity that you would consider easy or low level, assign 3 to 5 calories per minute. Give a moderate-level activity 6 to 10 calories per minute. If you're working hard, you get 11 to 15 calories per minute. If you've reached a level that could be categorized as super intensity, you rate 16 to 20 calories per minute. (A world-class marathoner or Nordic skier can reach energy expenditures approaching 20 calories per minute. That's Olympic intensity!)

Take the calories per minute assigned for a particular activity (based on your subjective rating) and multiply it by the number of minutes you spent exercising. (Rest between strength sets doesn't count—only those minutes spent active above resting levels. Most people overestimate the amount and intensity at which they do an activity, as well as underreport the amount of food they eat. Be honest!) This will give you a very rough estimate of the total calories you've used for a given activity. This rough estimation is based on a 155 pound body weight. If you weigh 120 pounds you'll burn fewer calories, and conversely, if you tip the scales at 200 pounds, you'll burn more calories per hour for any given effort.

Let's say you had a good 45-minute strength training session and you spent 30 minutes actually exercising. Thirty minutes multiplied by 6 calories per minute, or 180 total calories, is a good estimate. If you ran a 10-minute mile (6 mph) for 30 minutes, that represents a moderate pace and will net you about 10 calories per minute, or approximately 300 calories expended. Total formal activity calories for the day: 480.

Formula for Estimating Activity Energy Expenditure:
Calories per minute (for each given activity)
× Number of minutes spent exercising for each activity
= Formal exercise energy expenditure

Many factors influence the overall energy requirements of your body. Resting metabolic rate and physical activity represent the majority of total energy expenditure during a given day. Activity level, age, gender, size, weight, and

Table 10.1 Physical Activity Energy Expenditure

Level of Intensity	Examples	Calories per Minute
Low/easy	Weight training	6–10
Moderate	Jumping rope Jogging	11–15
High/difficult	Sprinting Fast rowing	16–20

body composition influence the final number of calories burned daily. To calculate exact daily caloric expenditure is beyond the capabilities of most scientific labs, let alone normal households!

Yet, it is possible to estimate resting metabolic rate and formal exercise energy requirements to give you a framework from which to formulate how many calories you should consume on a daily basis. If the numbers don't work (i.e., you gain weight and you're trying to lose some fat), you need to adjust your activity level or food intake. It is important to fine-tune the gross estimate to serve your exercising needs and accomplish your health and fitness goals. Table 10.1 gives the rate of calorie burn for activities of varying intensity.

3. Next, determine how many calories you use for daily activity that is separate from scheduled or formal exercise:

- If you are sedentary, add 20 to 40 percent of your RMR (found in step 1).
- If you are moderately active, add 40 to 60 percent of your RMR.
- If you are very active, add 60 to 80 percent of your RMR.

Worksheet for Estimating Your Daily Calorie Requirement

1.   Determine your RMR.

_____(Current body weight) × 10 =_____ (RMR)

2.   Estimate how many calories you need for your formal exercise each day.

Calories per minute (for each given activity) × Number of minutes spent exercising for each activity = Formal exercise energy expenditure

_____ (calories per minute) ×_____ (# of minutes exercising) = _____ (formal exercise energy expenditure)

_____ (calories per minute) × _____ (# of minutes exercising) = _____ (formal exercise energy expenditure)

_____ (calories per minute) × _____ (# of minutes exercising) = _____ (formal exercise energy expenditure)

To find total calories used for formal exercise, use the previous formula to calculate each formal exercise you participate in.

3. Determine how many calories you use for daily activity that is separate from scheduled or formal exercise:

- If you are sedentary, add 20 to 40 percent of your RMR (found in step 1).
- If you are moderately active, add 40 to 60 percent of your RMR.
- If you are very active, add 60 to 80 percent of your RMR.

_____ (percentage) × _____(RMR) = _____ (daily activity calories)

4. Add the answers from steps 1, 2, and 3 to compute this day's total calorie requirement:

_____ (RMR) + _____ (formal exercise calories) + _____ (daily activity calories) = _____ (calorie requirement for day)

Let's say you're on the high end of being moderately active.

$$60\% \times 1550 \text{ RMR} = \text{your daily activity calories}$$

$$0.6 \times 1550 \text{ RMR} = 930 \text{ daily activity calories}$$

4. Add the answers from steps 1, 2, and 3 to compute this day's total calorie requirement.

$$\begin{aligned}
&1550 \text{ calorie RMR} \\
&+ 480 \text{ formal exercise calories} \\
&+ 930 \text{ daily activity calories} \\
&= 2960 \text{ calorie requirement}
\end{aligned}$$

Steps 1, 3, and 4 are from Nancy Clark's *Sports Nutrition Guidebook: Eating to Fuel Your Active Lifestyle.* Champaign, IL: Human Kinetics, 1997.

Estimate Your Daily Caloric Range Using Lean Body Mass

To use this technique you must know your body fat percentage, which will allow you to calculate your lean body weight (LBW).

1. Multiply your body weight by your body fat percentage to get your body fat weight.

$$\text{Body weight} \times \text{Body fat percentage} = \text{Body fat weight}$$

Let's say you weigh 155 lbs. and your body fat percentage is 20.

$$155 \times 0.20 = 31 \text{ pounds of body fat}$$

2. Next, determine your lean body weight (LBW).

$$\text{Body weight} - \text{Body fat weight} = \text{LBW}$$
$$155 \text{ pounds} - 31 \text{ pounds} = 124 \text{ pounds of lean body weight (LBW)}$$

3. Once you have calculated LBW, multiply it by 16 to get the lower number in your daily caloric range.

$$124 \times 16 = 1984 \text{ calories}$$

4. Compute the upper number of the daily caloric range by adding 500 calories.

$$1984 \text{ calories} + 500 = 2484 \text{ calories}$$
$$\text{Daily caloric range: } 1984–2484 \text{ calories}$$

Fit and Healthy Lifestyles FitnessTrakker System manual, by Douglas Brooks and Derrick Pedranti, 1997.

Note that this calculation, when compared to the first technique (about 2960 daily calories required), is about 500 to 1,000 calories different, depending on whether you choose to use the high or low end of the range. This difference

Worksheet for Estimating Your Daily Caloric Range Using Lean Body Mass

1. Calculate body fat percentage.

_____ [body weight (lb.)] × _____ (body fat percentage) = _____ [body fat weight (lb.)]

2. Determine your LBW.

_____ (body weight) – (minus) _____ (body fat weight) = _____ (LBW)

3. Multiply LBW by 16 to determine the lower number in your daily caloric range.

____ (LBW) × 16 = _____ (lower number in daily caloric range)

4. Compute the upper number of the daily caloric range by adding 500 calories.

_____ (lower number in caloric range) + 500 calories = _____ (upper number caloric range)

5. Your daily calorie range is _____ (result from step 3, lower number in daily caloric range) to _____ (result from step 4, upper number in daily caloric range)

holds true even though both techniques for estimating daily calorie requirements used a person weighing 155 pounds. The first technique takes into account more variables (exercise, daily activity level) and may be a more accurate predictor of total daily caloric needs for very active people.

Now that you've computed your daily calorie requirements using one of two methods, heed this good advice: use common sense in adhering to these "guess-timations!" Consider these predictions for what they are—educated guesswork and general guides that can help you "ballpark" your daily calorie needs. You may need to fine-tune this number as your activities change or if you find you're not getting the results you want.

The number of calories you should be eating daily is not the whole calorie story. (I'll talk about the correct percentage of carbohydrate, fat, and protein later to help you create a balanced diet.) But, it's important to understand how to determine correct food portion size and read food labels. This will greatly impact the quantity and quality of food you eat.

Identify Correct Food Portion Size by Using a Food Scale

Not everyone can eat their cereal out of a trough like the legendary Ironman triathlete Dave Scott and still maintain performance and weight. (Dave probably expended about 5,000 to 6,000 calories per day in training.) I often use a food scale with my personal training clients to drive home the important issue of portion control. It is not a shock to me that a majority of my clients vastly *underestimate* the amount of food they eat. For example, many of my clients thought an acceptable serving from the fish, poultry, or meat group was anything set in front of them. Obviously, a 16-ounce steak is over five times the recommended three-ounce serving! I have asked clients to pour three to four ounces of cereal in a bowl (Dave probably poured the box in), and to their amazement the scale reveals anywhere from six to eight ounces.

By using the food scale you can learn quickly how to accurately judge serving sizes. The visual image of, for example, an ounce of cereal or three ounces of lean meat is a very powerful teaching tool. This approach has helped many of my clients who have struggled, not so much with poor food choices, but with simply consuming too much food. My clients jokingly refer to this syndrome as too much of a good thing. Once you get the picture you can stop measuring your food, or at least do it less often, because you have a visual frame of reference.

Realize that if you border on undereating, portions that are too small can also jeopardize your health, performance, and weight management goals. Eating too few calories can lead to fatigue, poor performance, and in extreme cases, eating disorders. If you think this situation applies to you, contact a registered dietitian and discuss your situation.

How to Read Food Labels

Although the food labels we see on all food produced in the United States are not as useful and easy to understand as they could be, they still can help you assess the food you are buying. The new labels can help you be more aware of fat intake, quickly see food portion or serving size, and identify what kinds of nutrients are present in the serving. Following is a description of the elements of the labels.

Serving Size

Serving size (see item 1 below) helps with realistic estimates of total caloric intake and keeping track of the number of servings of a particular food group. As mentioned earlier, a food scale is an effective teaching tool to learn serving size. Actually seeing a serving size on a scale will help you understand and see, for example, what a one-ounce serving looks like. This will help you accurately estimate appropriate portion or serving sizes.

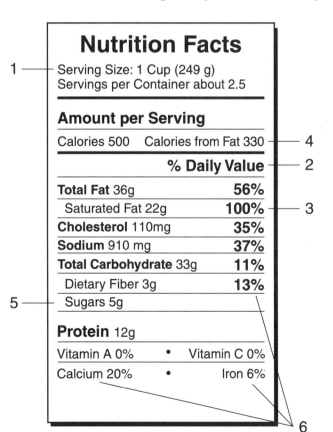

Percent Daily Value

The percent daily value column (item 2) tells you how much of the day's worth of fat, cholesterol, sodium, carbohydrate, dietary fiber, and sugar the food provides. If a food contains 20 percent or more of the daily value, whether fat or carbohydrate, it could be considered high in that nutrient. Low is probably no more than 5 percent.

Figure 10.1 The nutrition facts on food labels inform consumers of recommended serving sizes and daily values, and the amount of fats, sugars, calories, and vitamins and minerals in commercial products.

Saturated Fat

Because saturated fat (item 3) probably causes the most damage to your health, this particular percentage of the daily value is important to note. (Unfortunately, trans fat or hydrogenated oil, which is just as damaging, is not reported. If hydrogenated oil is the first item listed in the food product's ingredients, it's loaded with trans fat and you may want to limit your intake.)

Calories From Fat

Calories from fat (item 4) help you quickly see how much fat is in each serving of this particular food. In this example, 330 calories of each 500-calorie serving is from fat. If you divide 330 by 550, you can calculate that 60 percent of each serving is fat! Many experts recommend a daily fat intake of no more than 20 percent of total daily calories. This does not mean that you shouldn't eat this food (it's only *part* of your total daily calories), but it must be balanced with the overall daily intake.

Sugar

The FDA has not set a daily value for sugar (item 5) because health experts have not yet set a limit on how much should be eaten on a daily basis. Furthermore, this number is not very accurate because it does not contain all types of sugars. Limit intake of simple sugars whenever possible.

Percent Daily Values of Healthier Nutrients

The percent daily values (item 6) are based on a daily intake of 2,000 calories. This is very interesting because it allows you to compare the percent daily value for healthier nutrients (vitamins A and C, calcium and iron, and dietary fiber) against fat, sodium, and cholesterol.

KEY POINT

The information on food labels can be used to improve food selection and overall health.

The typical diet is high in sodium, cholesterol, saturated fat, and total calories. Research has documented that this type of diet greatly increases the risk of heart disease, stroke, diabetes, and some cancers. Moreover, a high fat intake will certainly not complement athletic performance. An aggressive recommendation (for optimal health) is to limit fat intake to about 40 to 50 grams per day. I have found that many of my clients find it easier to focus solely on fat gram intake than on the myriad of other diet variables when their focus is weight loss and personal health. Athletes who train hard need to prioritize carbohydrate intake, too. Daily sodium intake should be kept below 2,000 milligrams.

KNOWING WHAT TO EAT

It is no secret that neither consumers nor experts (even among themselves!) can agree on what constitutes optimal nutrition. Yet everyone wants instant gratification and results. At the forefront of that quick-fix mentality is the word *diet*. To me, a diet is usually associated with severe calorie restriction; deprivation; or some other extreme, unscientific approach. While a myriad of diets exist, including the Why Women Need Chocolate diet, the Zone Favorable High-Fat diet, Carbohydrate Addict's diet, the Fit for Life diet, the Eat Smart Think Smart diet, the Eat 'til You Puke and Still Lose Weight diet, and dozens more, believe me, a magical, quick-fix nutritional program does not exist. According to Kelly Brownell, director of the Center for Eating and Weight Disorders at Yale University, all of these diets have equally compelling testimonials from "pseudo experts" who believe, or want you to believe, that they have something new.

However, not all diets are bad. You have been hearing for years about low-fat diets. The premise is that by cutting down on the fat in your diet and replacing it with healthier choices, you can easily and automatically cut calories, lose weight, decrease your risk for a host of illnesses, and perform better. Some researchers believe that it doesn't matter *what* you eat as long as you cut total calories. Nevertheless, since fat has over twice the calories per gram as carbohydrate or protein, you can eat the same or larger *amount* of low-fat food and still take in fewer calories. Limiting fat intake is also a good idea to help prevent heart disease. Also, since muscles are fueled largely by carbohydrates, appropriate carbohydrate intake is important.

The sensible eating guidelines I offer my clients are always intermingled with ideas for low-fat eating. That is the basis of a healthy diet.

Ratio of Carbohydrates, Fats, and Protein

Most sport nutritionists (who are qualified and licensed as registered dietitians or RDs) recommend a daily training diet composed of about 60 to 65 percent carbohydrate, 20 to 25 percent fat (you'll take in more fat than you think because it's hidden in many foods, so shoot for the lower number—it's good for your heart), and 15 percent protein. If you're training hard, you should probably bump the carbohydrate intake up to 70 percent before an event (especially if it's an endurance event), or as your training dictates (e.g., you don't fully recover between workouts and can't shake that fatigued feeling). To raise your carbohydrate intake easily, cut the fat and increase your intake of starches, grains, and fruits (don't overload on simple sugars that come from fruit). In later sections I'll discuss why adequate carbohydrate intake is the most important factor in your performance and how you feel.

One of the best ways to determine the *amount* of carbohydrate, fat, and protein in your diet is to (1) determine your daily caloric intake based on total energy expenditure using one of the two methods described earlier in this chapter, and (2) calculate carbohydrate (multiply by 60 to 65 percent), fat (multiply by 20 to 25 percent), and protein (multiply by 15 percent) needs. Focus on ingesting enough carbohydrates. If you load your diet with starches, grains, cereals, pasta, and fruits, you won't go overboard on fats and protein.

Use the label-reading skills you learned earlier to help you gauge the amount (grams) of each nutrient you are putting into your body on a daily basis. Initially, it is important to track, calculate, and record this nutritional information by writing it down. Soon you'll become an expert at estimating and having an intuition for selecting the right balance of foods you eat each day. Don't

Table 10.2   Worksheet for Determining Carbohydrate, Fat, and Protein Ratios

Determine your daily caloric requirement. Using technique #1 for determining daily caloric requirement, my sample 155-pound person required almost 3,000 calories for that given day to support his exercise, activity, and basal metabolic requirements.

	Total daily calorie intake	Desired percent of each nutrient	Number of calories from daily intake	Number of calories in one gram of the nutrient	Number of grams of nutrient
Carbohydrate	3,000 calories	.65	3,000 × .65 = 1950 calories	4	1950 ÷ 4 = 487.5 grams
Fat	3,000 calories	.20	3,000 × .20 = 600 calories	9	600 ÷ 9 = 67 grams
Protein	3,000 calories	.15	3,000 × .15 = 450 calories	4	450 ÷ 4 = 112.5 grams

worry about being forever tied to recording your eating behavior. However, if you like the exactness and accountability of recording your nutritional intake, keep doing it. If you feel you've got it down and are seeing the results you want, it's still a good idea to jot down your intake periodically and calculate your percentages of carbohydrate, fat, and protein, just to make sure you're still on track.

An easy method for calculating carbohydrate intake is based on body weight only. Researcher Liz Applegate, PhD, determined that three to five grams of carbohydrate per pound of body weight accurately reflects your carbohydrate needs. Additionally, research supports taking in about 0.6 to 0.9 grams of protein per pound of body weight.

The upper end of the range of carbohydrate requirements (five grams per pound of body weight) reflects the carbohydrate needs for very active athletes. The lower end of the range (three grams per pound of body weight) is appropriate for an active person looking for the recommended carbohydrate intake of about 60 to 65 percent.

Table 10.3   Worksheet for Calculating Carbohydrate and Protein Needs per Pound of Body Weight

	Body weight (lb.)	Grams per pound of body weight	Body weight × grams of nutrient per pound	Grams required per pound of body weight
Carbohydrate	155 lb.	3–5 grams	155 × 3 = 465 g 155 × 5 = 775 g	465–775 grams
Protein	155 lb.	0.6–0.9 grams	155 × 0.6 = 93 g 155 × 0.9 = 139.5 g	93–139.5 grams

The protein recommendations (0.6 to 0.9 grams per pound of body weight) provide for a range of individual protein needs. It is important to note that these amounts are not minimal but provide a margin of safety as well. Individuals who have high protein needs include athletes who exercise intensely (endurance athletes and those doing strength training), people who consume too few carbohydrate calories (protein can be converted to sugar and used for energy instead of being used to build muscles and repair the body), untrained individuals just starting a strength/exercise program, and growing teenagers (they need protein for proper growth and activity). Having said that, excessive amounts of protein do not enhance any of these situations.

Even though heavier body weight requires greater absolute amounts (grams) of carbohydrate, fat, and protein, the percentages of each nutrient do not change!

Carbohydrate should form the foundation of every meal or snack you eat. Carbohydrates ultimately fuel your muscles. Without adequate intake, your training suffers, you feel stale, and the life and "spring" of your body slowly oozes away!

KEY POINT

Overtraining and that burned-out feeling can be caused by insufficient carbohydrate intake!

On the other hand, fat and protein provide important nutrients that enhance training and health. Don't go carbohydrate crazy. Too much of a good thing can harm you, too. It is important that you provide enough fat and protein in your diet to fuel optimal health and training response, and for a well-balanced diet.

Building Muscle Safely and Sensibly

When asked what the best way is to put on muscle, most people would respond, "Eat lots of protein!" or, "Drink shakes for extra calories!" Wrong! Calories, regardless of whether they are in the form of carbohydrate, fat (shakes are usually loaded with fat and extra calories), or protein do not automatically turn into muscle. A high-protein diet does not necessarily result in more muscle, since excess protein is not stored as muscle (any calories in excess of your daily caloric requirements will be stored as fat).

Although you do need extra calories if you're training hard, those calories should come predominantly from carbohydrate food sources. Carbohydrates are necessary to fuel your muscles so they can perform intense strength training (muscle-building) exercise and recover from hard effort. The stimulus for your muscles to grow larger (hypertrophy) comes from overloading them with correct and intense strength exercise, and not from overloading your body (including your kidneys) with too much protein.

Protein Sources

Your protein requirements can be met by eating two to three servings of protein-rich foods per day. This represents about four to six ounces of food that is rich in protein. If you question what three ounces of protein looks like, use a food scale to measure your next serving of tuna or poultry. Once you get this frame of reference, you're in business. Most Americans who eat a 16-ounce steak or half a chicken view this as a serving and move unknowingly well beyond their daily protein requirements. On the other hand, if you're always chewing on bagels, bread, plain pasta, vegetables, salads, and fruit, you can easily take in too little protein.

Excellent protein-rich foods (which contain important amino acids) include lean beef, fish (you'll find tuna, salmon, and swordfish here), chicken and turkey, peanut butter, tofu, canned beans, and low-fat dairy products. Don't forget to read the food label to determine the grams of protein each serving provides.

HOW TO EAT BEFORE, DURING, AND AFTER WORKOUTS

When and what you eat can dramatically affect your performance, your next workout, and how you feel. As discussed, appropriate carbohydrate, fat, and protein intake are important before and after intense, anaerobic training (such as sprints and strength training), but what you eat before, during, and after exercise also affects endurance-related performance.

Realize that one food that is another athlete's perfect match may not work for you. Even though certain types of foods may or may not work for you before, during, or after your workout, certain categories (carbohydrate, fat, and protein) of food are best eaten at specific times within your overall training schedule. The timing and type of nutrient to ingest is well defined by science. Within each nutrient category, you will have to decide what works best for your pre-exercise or precompetition meal. For example, in the category of carbohydrate, does a plain bagel or piece of toast, a banana, or cereal sit better in your stomach?

What to Eat Before Your Workout (and When!)

From a practical standpoint, what and when you eat can be influenced by the type of activity you perform (running and impact versus cycling) and how your body tolerates food intake prior to activity. However, science should also guide your decision.

Pre-exercise food intake can cause abdominal/intestinal discomfort and diarrhea. Nevertheless, it's important to your workout or competition. Following are some guidelines to help you manage the question, "Should I eat before I work out or compete?"

Pre-Exercise Nutrition Guidelines

1. Maintain a low-fat, high-carbohydrate diet on a daily basis. This will keep your glycogen (stored carbohydrate/sugar) stores in the muscles and liver at adequate levels.

2. Avoid foods high in fat and protein prior to working out or competing.

3. If you're exercising for less than an hour, common carbohydrate choices include bagels, plain or toasted bread, crackers, plain pasta, and bananas. Try different foods and find one or several that don't upset your stomach.

4. If you're exercising longer than an hour, try foods such as bananas, oatmeal, and apples because they have a low glycemic index. (While apples have a low glycemic index, you may want to experiment because the fructose may upset your stomach. Other low glycemic index foods are listed in the box on page 191.) Foods such as this will help fuel your performance as you exercise for longer periods of time.

5. Before you eat simple sugars (sodas, candies, and some sport drinks) or any foods with a high glycemic index within 15 to 120 minutes before a hard workout, experiment first. Some athletes experience a huge drop in blood sugar after such a fix. This leaves them feeling exhausted, lightheaded, and off their game. On the other hand, many athletes (and research confirms this) experience an improvement in performance.

To play it safe, consume your sweet snack about 5 to 10 minutes before you exercise. This time span is probably too short to allow insulin to be secreted from the pancreas into the bloodstream and draw your blood sugar down. When you start exercising, your body stops secreting insulin and you should be fine. Be sure to experiment with ingesting simple sugars before exercise to see how your body responds. The "sugar blues" can result in your feeling fatigued and irritable and may even cause your stomach to start rumbling. Avoid this quick sugar fix if you experience these or similar symptoms. If it works for you, great! Research is on your side! If you can stomach it, it will improve performance. To escape the need for a quick fix, try eating more food two to four hours before your next workout or competition.

Pre-exercise nutrition can help you maintain even levels of blood sugar and prevent early fatigue. The right foods taken at the right time can calm your stomach by neutralizing stomach acids and keep you from feeling starved. Carbohydrate fuel eaten well in advance of your workout can fuel your performance as exercise intensity dictates, as a result of glycogen being stored in the muscle or liver. Foods (especially carbohydrates with a low glycemic index rating) eaten about an hour before your workout are broken down enough to be used as fuel, and they will continue to be metabolized throughout the exercise session, but do little to replenish glycogen stores. To replenish glycogen stores, load up after exercise (see the section "What to Eat After Your Workout") and three to four hours before exercise, and maintain your daily high-carbohydrate diet.

What to Eat During Your Workout

Most people who exercise longer than 30 minutes can tolerate small amounts of food in their stomachs, similar to the types discussed in the previous section. Moderate- to even high-intensity endurance activity still allows for food to digest and you do exercise more effectively. However, if you're doing an all-out effort, you may get the opportunity to revisit what you ate!

If your endurance exercise lasts longer than 60 minutes, your nutritional challenge becomes a management game that attempts to preserve a balance in your fluid and carbohydrate reservoirs. Your fluid intake must match your sweat loss (you lose water through breathing and sweating), and your carbohydrate intake helps maintain stamina by providing energy and sustaining blood sugar levels. Every hour of endurance exercise requires about 100 to 300

Glycemic Index of Some Popular Foods

A glycemic index rating for a food is determined by its ability to contribute glucose (sugar) to the bloodstream. For example, eat honey and your bloodstream will quickly become loaded with sugar. Quick entry of a sugar into the bloodstream is desirable if you're already exercising or recovering from exercise. Low or moderate glycemic index foods before exercise are preferable when performing exercise longer than an hour because they provide a food source for sustained energy needs. It will be used as you exercise rather than being dumped into your bloodstream immediately. High glycemic index foods stimulate insulin production, which can be stored as glycogen, but can also cause your blood sugar to drop lower than your pre-meal level.

You cannot rate a food as high or low glycemic based solely on its classification as a simple or complex carbohydrate. You might think that an apple (low glycemic index and simple carbohydrate) would have a similar index as watermelon (high glycemic index and simple carbohydrate). Use the table below to decide which foods are appropriate for your needs.

Food*	GI	Food	GI
High		Popcorn	55
		Corn	55
Glucose	100	Sweet potato	54
Potato, baked	85	Pound cake, Sara Lee	54
Corn flakes	84	Banana, overripe	52
Rice cakes	82	Peas, green	48
Potato, microwaved	82	Bulgur	48
Jelly beans	80	Baked beans	48
Vanilla wafers, Nabisco	77	Rice, white parboiled	47
Cheerios	74	Lentil soup	44
Cream of Wheat, instant	74	Orange	43
Graham crackers	74	All-Bran cereal	42
Honey	73	Spaghetti (no sauce)	41
Watermelon	72	Pumpernickel bread	41
Bagel, Lender's white	72	Apple juice, unsweetened	41
Bread, white	70		
Bread, whole wheat	69 (65-75)	**Low**	
Shredded wheat	69		
Soft drink, Fanta	68	Apple	36
Mars Bar	68	Pear	36
Grape-Nuts	67	PowerBar	30-35
Stoned wheat thins	67	Chocolate milk	34
Cream of Wheat, regular	66	Fruit yogurt, low-fat	33
Couscous	65	Chick-peas	33
Table sugar (sucrose)	65	PR Bar	33
Raisins	64	Lima beans, frozen	32
Oatmeal	61 (42-75)	Split peas, yellow	32
Ice cream	61 (36-80)	Milk, skim	32
		Apricots, dried	31
Moderate		Green beans	30
Muffin, bran	60	Lentils	29
Bran Chex	58	Kidney beans	27
Orange juice	57	Milk, whole	27
Potato, boiled	56	Barley	25
Rice, white long grain	56	Grapefruit	25
Rice, brown	55	Fructose	23

*Amount based on 50 grams of carbohydrate per serving

Foods with a high glycemic response have a value above 60; foods with a moderate glycemic response have a value between 40 to 60; and foods with a low glycemic response have a value less than 40.

Data from food companies and K. Foster-Powell and J. Brand Miller, 1995, "International tables of glycemic index," Am J Clin Nutr 62: 871S-893S.

Reprinted, with permission, from Nancy Clark, 1997. *Nancy Clark's Sport Nutrition Guidebook,* 2nd ed. (Champaign, IL: Human Kinetics).

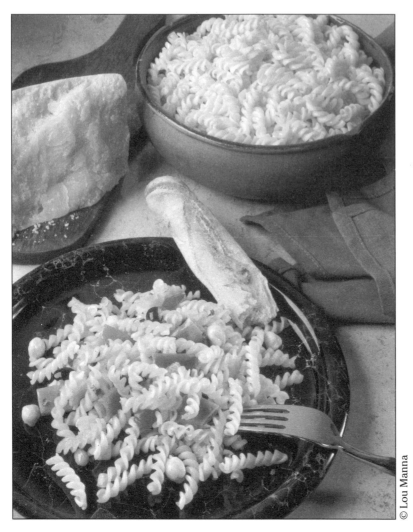

© Lou Manna

Foods high in carbohydrates such as pasta will ensure your muscles have the fuel they need.

calories of carbohydrates (or more exact, 0.5 grams of carbohydrates per pound of body weight).

A person weighing 155 pounds (155 × 0.5) would require 77.5 grams of carbohydrate every hour. Physiologically, your body is indifferent to whether food is in the form of a liquid or a solid. Runners, probably because of impact and jarring, seem to prefer liquids, whereas people who participate in activities that have little impact seem to use either depending on how well the type of food sits with them. For example, it's easy to carry and eat solid food when cycling, and there is no jarring to wreak havoc on your intestinal system. Twelve 4-ounce gulps of a sport drink that provides 25 calories per 4-ounce serving would give you an hourly carbohydrate intake of 300 calories. Some combination of sport drinks, sport bars, bananas, Fig Newtons (my personal favorite), and so on, and plain water can provide the necessary nutrients. Test and try out various options. You'll find a favorite that you swear by!

> **KEYPOINT**
>
> You cannot be competitive at longer durations without feeding while you exercise. Not only will you perform better, you'll feel great and enjoy the experience.

What to Eat After Your Workout (and When!)

This depends on whether you're a recreational exerciser who trains regularly or on a demanding, hard-core training program. If you work out three to five times per week at moderate to hard levels of effort and optimal performance is not one of your training goals, your glycogen stores can be replenished with a regular diet that is high in carbohydrate. If you practice twice a day, are competing two to three times per week in a competitive basketball or volleyball league, and work out in the gym, pay close attention to your recovery diet.

Athletes often fail to follow a proper recovery diet because they are unaware of its importance to their next day training/performance, are not hungry or too tired after the event/workout, or say they don't have the time. Make the time and prioritize this important aspect of your training program. It requires little forethought and is easy to do.

If you're training hard and often, you should be concerned with fluid replacement immediately after exercising to get ready for your next workout. Immediately upon cessation (and of course you should be hydrating during your workout or competition) of the exercise, begin to replace sweat/fluid losses with juices, foods high in water, sport drinks, soft drinks (nondiet drinks are OK for supplying carbohydrates, but provide virtually zero vitamins and minerals), and water.

Your first round of carbohydrate feeding should begin within 15 minutes after you stop exercising. If you wait longer than that, your glycogen stores will not be replenished as quickly. You need about 300 calories within two hours of finishing your exercise and should begin taking them in within 15 minutes of stopping. Carbohydrate-rich foods and beverages are the right food choice for recovery. Follow this initial feeding with about 300 additional carbohydrate calories every two hours thereafter for six to eight hours. In total, this represents three to four 300-calorie carbohydrate feedings over six to eight hours. A 12-ounce can of soda and a banana is all that it takes to provide your first 300 calories! After hard and sustained exercise, your body will crave these calories!

It's also a good idea to mix a little protein with your carbohydrate recovery foods. Protein, like carbohydrate, stimulates the production of insulin (a hormone), which helps herd blood glucose into the muscles to enhance glycogen replacement. Lean meat and low-fat milk are good examples. But don't go overboard. More is not better. Maintain your protein needs for muscle growth and cellular repair/production by keeping your protein intake at 15 percent of your daily calorie intake.

KEY POINT

After exercise, your priorities are carbohydrate and fluid replenishment.

Sport Drinks and Water Intake

You probably can't drink enough water before and after exercise, as long as you can tolerate it and have a chance to eliminate before you exercise. At a minimum, you should drink three to four ounces (a good-sized gulp) of water every 10 to 15 minutes during exercise. If you're exercising hard, you may require eight ounces of water every 15 to 20 minutes. To determine if you're taking in enough fluid to match your sweat losses, weigh yourself before and after each workout. Your after-workout weight should match your pre-exercise weight. If you're drinking enough water, your urine will be pale yellow or almost clear throughout the day, and there will be lots of it. Different environmental conditions and exercise intensities will require more or less fluid intake.

Sport drinks are designed to keep or raise your fluid and glycogen (carbohydrate) levels back up to pre-exercise levels. Some drinks also contain electrolytes (minerals) such as potassium and sodium since you lose these minerals when you sweat. Usually, a sport drink isn't an important consideration unless you exercise for at least an hour. In this case, your primary need is for water, not sugar or minerals. Additionally, a sport energy drink will replace most of the calories you use in a half-hour workout. To competitive athletes this is not important, but if one of your goals is to lose weight, stick with an energy drink called water!

Follow the guidelines for food intake before, during, and after workouts when considering the use of a commercial sport drinks. Remember, these are primarily carbohydrate (sugar) solutions that are weak (4 to 8 percent solutions that provide about 40 to 80 calories per eight ounces and work well when taken during exercise) or very concentrated (read this as "sweet and best taken as a recovery drink after exercise"). There is nothing magical about them, though they can be effective and convenient. You can dilute soft drinks or juices to this same weak solution of about 40 to 80 calories per eight ounces. A proper and balanced diet, along with using the guidelines for ingesting solid or liquid food before, during, and after exercise, can provide all of your nutrient needs regardless of whether you choose to use a commercial sport drink.

> ### KEY POINT
>
> Training without proper fluid intake does not toughen you. This habit simply makes you better at training when you're dehydrated and nowhere near your top performance capabilities.

Steps to Help You Eat Right

Now that you know what and when to eat, here are a few steps to follow that can help you sensibly change old eating habits.

Empower Yourself

Confidence, support, and a realistic approach are the key ingredients to healthy eating habits, weight control, and better performance. Two empowerment tools discussed in this chapter, label reading and learning food portion control with the food scale, will give you skills that will help you eat smart most of the time. Additionally, stress to yourself the theme of moderation. There is no need to be obsessed with food. Period! This is ultimately counterproductive. Keep the focus on health, feeling good, and performing better. Give yourself some slack and be more compassionate and patient with your progress and effort.

Phase in Behavior Change

Health, fitness, and athletic performance can be greatly impacted with small changes. Total cholesterol, LDL cholesterol (bad cholesterol), and triglycerides (fat in your blood) significantly drop (and HDL, or good, cholesterol significantly rises) every time you lose five pounds through diet and exercise. Knocking off five fat-pounds will help you run faster with less effort and stress on your joints. In one study, 60 percent of people with high blood pressure were able to discontinue their blood pressure medication after losing 10 pounds. Whether you're eating smart for health, fitness, or performance you'll receive benefits in all areas.

Transition to Healthy Food Choices

Evolving to healthier eating is very rewarding. However, remember that tastes are learned. Although some experts would argue that it's easier to make a complete change to a more wholesome diet—vegetables, grains, fruits, and legumes —I believe a moderate approach works the best. For example, replace high-fat dairy products with low-fat options before proceeding to nonfat sources. Another progression might be to eat meat less often and purchase cuts that are lowest in fat rather than completely eliminating it from the diet.

Practice Healthful Eating Habits

Drink more fluids and eat lots of fruits, vegetables, legumes, and grains instead of fat-free cakes and cookies loaded with "fake fat" and sugar. Reduce the intake of refined carbohydrates—which include white flour, white sugar, and white rice, to name a few— by choosing whole-grain products and natural sweeteners such as fruits, juices, and syrup. Reduce red meat, poultry, and fish. Limit hydrogenated oils or trans fat (be sure to read labels); they raise blood cholesterol as much as saturated fat. Gradually reduce both butter and margarine in your diet. Switch to nonfat or low-fat versions of prepared foods and dairy products.

Calculate Accurate Calorie Needs

While you should not adopt an inflexible approach to calorie counting, you need to have some sense of portion control and total daily caloric intake. Learn to compute your daily calories and read labels to get a feel for your daily caloric intake without going overboard toward a rigid calorie-counting regimen. You will quickly learn, for example, that not all single servings are the same. An eight-ounce serving of nonfat milk carries with it about 90 calories, whereas an eight-ounce serving of whole milk contains about 150 calories and more fat.

Consume Calories Evenly Throughout the Day

When the typical diet is analyzed, most of the daily caloric intake is consumed at night. Today's social patterns encourage a light or skipped breakfast, quick lunch, and late dinner, with overconsumption at this evening meal. Calories are best consumed throughout the day to optimize alertness, energy, and the caloric needs required for basic metabolic maintenance and daily physical activity. Continually eating or grazing throughout the day may not be the best idea, but three to five solid meals and low-fat nutritional snacks, such as fruit, may work best.

Eat a Low-Fat Diet

Here's a list of suggestions to help you:

1. Read food labels consistently and carefully.
2. Order all toppings and salad dressings on the side. This allows you to control the amount you use. Ask for light, low-fat, or nonfat options. If low-fat options are not available, dressings and toppings can be mixed with vinegar and lemon juice.
3. Reduce the use of cooking oils and oil-based salad dressings. Using Dijon mustard and nonfat plain yogurt is a great substitute for an oil-based salad dressing.

4. Limit your intake of baked goods that are high in fat. Cookie, pie, and doughnut calories are often at least 50 percent fat.

5. Replace mayonnaise or butter on your sandwiches with mustard. Eat bread plain.

6. Instead of using margarine, butter, or regular sour cream on your baked potato, use nonfat yogurt or nonfat sour cream.

7. Instead of frying food, bake, boil, or poach it.

8. Sauté food in a low-fat broth or small amount of olive oil. Avoid using solid fats.

9. Use low-fat or nonfat yogurt and cottage cheese and either skim (nonfat) or one percent fat milk.

10. Purchase lean cuts of meat and trim any visible fat.

11. Buy chicken and turkey without the skin or remove the skin before eating.

12. Buy ground beef only if it is labeled as 96 percent fat-free. Don't be fooled by "extra-lean ground beef."

13. For dessert, try sorbet, sherbet, nonfat or low-fat frozen yogurt, and fresh fruit.

14. Add water or seltzer to dilute juices and cut calories. Recognize that juices are a food and can add significant calories to your total daily intake.

15. When eating out, in general, order vegetarian, seafood, or poultry dishes instead of beef or pork. Order side dishes that are filling yet low in fat, such as rice. Don't forget that alcoholic beverages count about the same as fat calories. In movie theaters, request air-popped popcorn.

> ### KEY POINT
>
> It is not necessary to label fat as the enemy. Although a low-fat diet is essential to optimal performance and personal health, too little fat leads to an unbalanced nutrition program that is counterproductive to your training goals.

MONITORING YOUR EATING HABITS

While you should be conscious about what you eat, tracking what you put into your mouth doesn't have to be as complex as cellular physiology. In fact, using the few simple calculations that you learned in this chapter requires little time and can help you eat smart and be accountable. And you won't be tied to the math work forever.

Monitor your nutrition program by calculating daily calorie intake for at least several weeks. Use your daily calorie requirement to figure your daily carbohydrate needs as 60 to 65 percent, fat as 20 to 25 percent, and protein as 15 percent of your daily calorie requirement. Use a food scale to help you identify correct food portion sizes, and learn to read labels so you can keep track of how many grams of carbohydrate, fat, and protein you are taking in each day toward your allotted percentages.

Even after you become good at accurately estimating daily calorie requirements and taking in the right amount of carbohydrate, fat, and protein, recalculate periodically to keep yourself honest, adjusted to changes in your program, and on target!

Quick Index:

PART III

Your Training Programs

11 Muscle Endurance and Maximum Strength

Develop maximal strength and you will shape your body! Develop maximal strength and you will change how you look! Develop maximal strength and you will increase muscle size! As you lay the foundation for progressing to maximal strength development, you will tone your muscles and develop an important base of muscular strength/endurance.

This periodized program first helps you develop muscular endurance (shaping, toning, body-shaping—call it what you want) and then progresses you toward optimal strength development and size gains. In addition to having fun, you'll see great results and your mind and body will feel fresh. So go ahead, get started and experience the results of a periodized strength program.

OVERVIEW OF THE PLAN

Each phase of this 16-week program is four weeks long. Before you jump into this training program, write down your goals and evaluate your current level of fitness.

If your goal is to shape and tone your muscles rather than develop maximal size and strength, you will maintain your strength fitness by following the guidelines in the first two phases. If you're looking to increase muscle size, take on phases III and IV. Phases I and II prepare you for the high-intensity training you'll experience in phases III and IV, as well as for the high-intensity techniques found in chapter 12.

If you've already laid your strength training foundation by training for at least four weeks, doing 8 to 10 exercises per workout, performing 15 to 20 reps to fatigue, and lifting two to three times per week, you can start at phase II, or week 5 of this periodized strength program. As the program progresses, the training becomes harder.

Before getting started, I'll describe the data you'll put on the workout sheets.

- **Exercise order:** Choose at least 10 to 12 exercises that target all of the major muscle groups. Refer to chapter 7 for 15 of the best strength exercises that challenge all of the major muscles of the body.

- **Number of workouts per week:** Place one day of rest/recovery between each strength workout day. You can still train the cardiovascular component and/or stretch on these off strength days.

- **Number of sets/reps:** Although the number of sets and reps should be followed closely, they are not written in stone. The progression from week to week builds in some flexibility, but feel free to modify if you're not on top of your game.

- **Weight used:** The amount of weight you use is determined by the repetition goal. Regardless of whether the goal is to complete 20 or 6 reps, and independent of the type of strength training equipment, select a resistance that allows you to complete the target number of reps (or end within a given range of reps) with good form before reaching muscle fatigue.

- **Movement speed:** How much time you will spend on each movement. For example a 2:4 ratio represents two seconds lifting and four seconds lowering. If you're ever in doubt about movement speed, err on the side of going slower. Control, control, control!

- **Recovery time between sets:** To make the most of your time, use active recovery (stretch or exercise another body part while you recover from a given exercise). If you don't feel fully recovered after the allotted recovery duration, take more time.

Phase I: Muscular Endurance

Phase I of your periodized strength program lasts four weeks. The first two weeks consist of light to moderate workouts. This allows for a progressive adaptation to strength loads so that muscles, tendons, and ligaments can become stronger with less chance of being injured. After two weeks, the workouts consist of light, moderate, and heavy training resistance (higher repetition numbers reflect light loads, while lower numbers represent heavier resistance). See table 11.1.

Generally, as you become stronger you can perform more exercises or sets of repetitions, train more frequently, and take shorter rest periods between sets. All of these training variables are manipulated in each four-week phase of

Table 11.1 Phase I: Muscle Endurance
Length of phase: Four weeks

Goals: Develop general muscle strength and endurance fitness base; prepare for increasingly harder workouts

Week 1			
Workout	Number of sets	Number of reps	Recovery time between sets (minutes)
Workout 1	1	20	2
Workout 2	1	20	2
Week 2			
Workout	Number of sets	Number of reps	Recovery time between sets (minutes)
Workout 1	1—2	20	1
Workout 2	2	20	2
Workout 3 (optional)	1—2	20	1
Week 3			
Workout	Number of sets	Number of reps	Recovery time between sets (minutes)
Workout 1	2	15	2
Workout 2	1—2	15	2
Workout 3	2	15	2
Week 4			
Workout	Number of sets	Number of reps	Recovery time between sets (minutes)
Workout 1	2	15	1
Workout 2	3	15	2
Workout 3	2	15	1

your 16-week program. These changes accommodate your new gains in fitness and provide new challenges (overload). You'll keep getting stronger and building more muscle, and you'll gain these results safely.

Phase II: Muscular Strength and Hypertrophy (Level 1)

Phase II of your periodized strength program lasts four weeks. With further increases in volume (reps, sets) and intensity (resistance), this phase is designed to result in an even greater stimulus for increased muscle size and strength gains. More emphasis is placed on distinct light, moderate, and heavy training sessions. Recovery time and number of reps decrease as this phase progresses, making your training harder and providing a greater stimulus for increased muscle size and strength gains. See table 11.2.

Phase III: Muscular Strength and Hypertrophy (Level 2)

Phase III of your periodized strength program lasts four weeks and is designed to present a new training stimulus that will continue to further your strength

Table 11.2 Phase II: Muscular Strength and Hypertrophy (Level 1) Length of phase: Four weeks

Goals: Increase muscular strength and size

Week 5			
Workout	Number of sets	Number of reps	Recovery time between sets (minutes)
Workout 1	3	20	1
Workout 2	3–4	15	2
Workout 3	3	15	1
Week 6			
Workout	Number of sets	Number of reps	Recovery time between sets(minutes)
Workout 1	3–4	20	1
Workout 2	3–4	15	2
Workout 3	3	12	2
Week 7			
Workout	Number of sets	Number of reps	Recovery time between sets (minutes)
Workout 1	4	20	1
Workout 2	2–4	15	2
Workout 3	4	12	2
Week 8			
Workout	Number of sets	Number of reps	Recovery time between sets (minutes)
Workout 1	3	12	1–2
Workout 2	2	15	1
Workout 3	3–4	12	1–2

and muscle size gains. During this phase, the biggest emphasis will be on lowering the number of repetitions (see table 11.3). Heavier resistance will provide yet another new stimulus to promote strength gains. Since you're using heavier resistance that may require more recovery from each set of exercise than I've allotted in the chart, allow more time when necessary so that you're fully recovered. A full recovery allows you to lift safely with heavier weights. During the last week of this phase (week 12), overall work is reduced slightly. This gives you a little recovery time before you jump into the last strength phase. Don't feel guilty. Phase IV (beginning week 13) will give you plenty of opportunity to work very hard as repetitions continue to decrease.

Phase IV: Optimizing Hypertrophy and Strength

The last phase of your periodized strength program lasts four weeks and is designed to put the finishing touches on your strength program. In this phase, the number of reps is decreased even further. Longer rest periods are used because this approach requires hard effort, which in turn requires longer

Table 11.3 Phase III: Muscular Strength and Hypertrophy (Level 2) Length of phase: Four weeks

Goals: Significantly increase muscular strength and size

Week 9			
Workout	Number of sets	Number of reps	Recovery time between sets (minutes)
Workout 1	3	12	1
Workout 2	2	10	1–2
Workout 3	3	12	1
Week 10			
Workout	Number of sets	Number of reps	Recovery time between sets (minutes)
Workout 1	3	10	1–2
Workout 2	3–4	12	1
Workout 3	3	10	1–2
Week 11			
Workout	Number of sets	Number of reps	Recovery time between sets (minutes)
Workout 1	3–4	10	1
Workout 2	3	8	1–2
Workout 3	3	10	1
Week 12			
Workout	Number of sets	Number of reps	Recovery time between sets (minutes)
Workout 1	3–4	10	1
Workout 2	3	10	1
Workout 3	2	10	1

recoveries between exercises to maintain a consistent level of exertion (meaning you need to be able to complete the assigned number of reps) from exercise to exercise. See table 11.4.

You can create and record your own periodized strength workouts on the reproducible form found on page 206.

DO HIGH REPETITIONS WORK?

As you consider strength training program design options and periodization choices, it is important to make choices that help you attain your goals. Muscular endurance is defined as the ability to sustain repeated contractions without undue fatigue over a longer and longer time period (for example, about 12 to 20 reps). As you become stronger, your muscles are more resistant to fatigue and you can perform more reps at a given resistance. As reps increase beyond about 20 (nothing magical here, this number just represents an estimation), the movement starts to resemble the overload definition for cardiovascular conditioning (continuous, rhythmic movement).

Table 11.4 Phase IV: Optimizing Hypertrophy and Strength
Length of phase: Four weeks

Goals: Maximize muscle strength and hypertrophy increases

Week 13			
Workout	Number of sets	Number of reps	Recovery time between sets (minutes)
Workout 1	3	8	2
Workout 2	2	10	1
Workout 3	3–4	8	2
Week 14			
Workout	Number of sets	Number of reps	Recovery time between sets (minutes)
Workout 1	3	8	2
Workout 2	2	6	2–3
Workout 3	3	8	2
Week 15			
Workout	Number of sets	Number of reps	Recovery time between sets (minutes)
Workout 1	3	6	2–3
Workout 2	3	6	2–3
Workout 3	3	6	2–3
Week 16			
Workout	Number of sets	Number of reps	Recovery time between sets (minutes)
Workout 1	3–4	6	2–3
Workout 2	3	6	2–3
Workout 3	3–4	6	2–3

However, *do not* interpret this statement to imply that significant cardiovascular conditioning takes place with high-repetition resistance training schemes. Actually, the load generally does not engage enough muscle mass to generate significant cardiovascular training effect, even if you're doing lots of reps.

For increases in strength, you have to present an intensity to the body's musculature to which it is unaccustomed on a regular and progressive basis. This type of intensity is necessary to stimulate the cellular machinery for muscle growth, or to stimulate your nervous system to become better at activating previously dormant muscle fibers. For the beginning to conditioned exerciser, that means about 6 to 20 repetitions to muscular fatigue. The number works as well for older adults as it does for athletes, since it does not define an absolute weight. Instead, the amount of weight lifted reflects the current strength level of the individual and is determined by the amount of resistance that creates muscle fatigue between 6 and 20 reps.

High-repetition schemes are usually highly ineffective in promoting any kind of health and fitness gains; they do not produce significant gains in muscular strength and endurance over an extended period of time and have little to no effect on cardiovascular conditioning. Repetitions that are redundantly high can lead to overuse injuries, not to mention lack of results and frustration.

Table 11.5 Strength Training Workout Sheet

#	Exercises	Weekly sets/reps	Set	Day 1 1	Day 1 2	Day 1 3	Day 1 4	Day 2 1	Day 2 2	Day 2 3	Day 2 4	Day 3 1	Day 3 2	Day 3 3	Day 3 4
1			Wt.												
			Reps												
2			Wt.												
			Reps												
3			Wt.												
			Reps												
4			Wt.												
			Reps												
5			Wt.												
			Reps												
6			Wt.												
			Reps												
7			Wt.												
			Reps												
8			Wt.												
			Reps												
9			Wt.												
			Reps												
10			Wt.												
			Reps												

Comments _____

Phase _____ Week _____

Date _____

DESIGNING STRENGTH PROGRAMS THAT WORK

Are you focusing on elite or advanced strength? Are you an older adult or looking to invest a minimal amount of time yet still see significant strength gains? There is much confusion surrounding the number of reps and sets and the amount of resistance, or load, one should use with varying populations. The confusion is related to physiological responses to loads (resistance) put on the musculature of the body. By looking at two case study strength programs, one of an Olympic-style lifter and the other of a 38-year-old adult, I hope to clear up some of the confusion and seemingly contradictory recommendations.

Many proposed programs are based on anecdotal and empirical evidence. Often the results are linked to the specific system of reps, sets, and loads that is popularized, when in fact the reasons for the results have little to do with the actual regimen and its supposed magical features.

Case Study 1: Olympic Lifter

John is an Olympic lifter. Olympic lifting is a competitive sport that involves two technical and explosive lifting movements known as the "clean and jerk" and the "snatch." John maintains high levels of muscle strength, joint flexibility, and neuromuscular coordination. He has had years of specialized training.

His goals are based on the demands of the sport: to accomplish maximal strength development and 1-RM lifts. You'll see how this is represented in the sample program below, which shows a typical protocol for Olympic lifters.

Examples of exercises that John uses include clean-and-jerk lifts, snatch lifts, bench presses, squat variations, dead lifts, jerks from the rack, military presses, shoulder shrugs, back hyperextensions, and abdominal and leg curls.

Since the requirements of the sport dictate the training regimen, most of John's training is centered around preparing for the required lifts. Some of these exercises are high risk, but they are what the sport demands. When John's goal is increasing strength, he does one to six reps and uses a variety of exercises. When he is training for overall program goals and practicing technique, he sometimes must practice the exact competition lifts with 1-RM lifts because this replicates competition and specificity, whereas other times he will lighten the weight and perfect his lifting technique with higher RMs, such as 7 to 10 reps.

Strength Training Program for an Olympic Lifter

Goal	Maximum strength/power development.
Repetitions (resistance/load)	1- to 6-RM (also use higher RMs to practice lifting technique and to periodize program).
Sets	Three to six sets for each exercise.
Rest/recovery	Two to five minutes between each set for full energy system recovery.
Frequency	One to three sessions per day and four to six days per week.

Case Study 2: Middle-Aged Adult

Janet is 38 years old and participates in a regular walking program. She has just begun a muscular strength and endurance conditioning program. She was motivated by reports that resistance training can positively affect osteoporosis, increase metabolism and calorie burning, influence posture, and help her maintain her physical independence. Janet's program resembles the sample program shown below.

Exercise examples for Janet include pressing movements (dumbbell presses, cable presses), pulling movements (dumbbell rows, rowing machine), overhead presses, lat pull-downs, leg extensions, leg curls, balance training (closing one's eyes while standing on one leg on a spongy floor surface) for leg abductors/adductors, leg presses, squats, lunges, and abdominal and back exercises.

Traditionally, clients such as Janet are encouraged to perform three sets. Performing one to two sets with the appropriate overload is more time efficient and will probably get her the results she's looking for. Although exercising three days per week might be better (although not significantly), exercising twice per week may be advantageous because it increases compliance (you stick with it because it doesn't take much time) and interest.

Notice that the amount of weight being lifted is not listed for John or Janet (you must determine your own weights for this chapter's periodized program, too). The amount of resistance is determined by an appropriate resistance that fatigues the muscle within the stated repetition goal range. The key to strength development is high-intensity effort. Resistance (load) should be sufficient to fatigue the target muscle group within about 30 to 90 seconds after the exercise is begun.

Rather than comparing apples (John) to oranges (Janet), let's compare oranges to oranges. Janet's friend Paul, who is also 38, has joined in the same fitness pursuit as Janet. Since their goals are similar, their exercise programs

Strength Training Program for a Middle-Aged Adult (Who is Time-Crunched!)

Goal	To optimize strength gains with minimal time investment using 8 to 10 strength exercises that target all of the major muscles. (This program will not maximize strength and hypertrophy gains, but doing two workouts per week will give you 75 to 80 percent of the strength gains you'd ever see, compared to working out more often and performing more sets of exercise!)
Repetitions (resistance/load)	During introduction to training, 15- to 20-RM to muscular fatigue; progress to 12- to 15-RM. After three to six months of training, progress to 6- to 12-RM to muscular fatigue if your goal is to optimize strength and size development.
Sets	During introduction to training, one per exercise; after four to six weeks of training, one to two per exercise.
Rest/recovery	Twenty seconds to 2 minutes between sets. Use active recovery to minimize downtime.
Frequency	One 25- to 30-minute session per day and two days per week.

will be the same. But this does not mean they will lift an identical amount of weight. For example, after Paul has trained for eight weeks, both may fatigue at 10-RM. However, Janet may use a 12-pound weight for a given lift, while Paul—who joined the program later and has not been training as long—may use an 8-pound weight to reach muscle fatigue at 10-RM. Conversely, Paul might be lifting more weight for the given lift even though both fatigue at 10-RM and Janet has been lifting longer. It all comes down to working out at the right number of reps to fatigue, regardless of absolute weight being lifted.

When would John or Janet change their programs? For John, the Olympic lifter who wants to be competitive, there is really no flexibility. The demands of the sport determine how John will train. Periodization will create the main variation.

Janet's program, on the other hand, can be as varied as her needs and wants. Her results are based on personal goals, not on sport performance. Even if she is physiologically ready to increase the weight load, only her interest in doing so will prompt her to change the program.

KEY POINT

When you're ready for a change, use your knowledge to execute the change and determine its appropriateness according to your goals and interest.

MAKING THE MOST OF YOUR STRENGTH WORKOUTS

No two people are likely to respond in the same manner to a given training program. Make sure you keep accurate lifting records (reps, sets, resistance, order of exercise, and periodization planning program) so that you can determine the combinations that best stimulate your mind and body. Your records and self-testing (e.g., body fat and strength tests) will help determine the changes your program needs and whether or not it is effective. Strength training program design is a process that demands constant evaluation, manipulation, and change.

Quick Index:

12 High-Intensity Strength Training

Without a doubt, high-intensity strength training is fierce and concentrated and requires focus. However, for those who are prepared and motivated to move their stalled strength training program (called a training plateau) to the next level, this chapter is exactly where you need to start. Training plateaus occur when your rate of training improvement slows down. This can result from the indefinite use of one training program approach or simply because you've been a dedicated strength trainer for a long time and your body needs new stimulation.

High-intensity strength training provides a way to train harder without increasing your workout times. In other words, you can increase intensity without doing more, but you will be working harder and getting results. High-intensity training techniques require greater muscular effort and place more intense physical demands on your muscles. These techniques push you to a greater degree of fatigue.

In theory, because you don't allow the fatigued motor units a chance to recover and be used again in the exercise you're currently performing, this type of training recruits muscle fibers (motor units) that are not normally challenged. Manipulating the amount of resistance you work against, eliminating recovery upon reaching momentary muscle fatigue and performing more reps while fatigued, and controlling how fast you move the weight (speed of movement) are commonly used methods to move strength training into the high-intensity realm. When using high-intensity strength training techniques, expect results, because you will get them! You will have also earned them!

If you're very fit and highly motivated, you can use one of the following techniques, but first make sure your goals are in line with these approaches. They require a good strength conditioning base and high degree of physical effort and are associated with physical discomfort (you're really pushing it here!). High-intensity training requires more recovery (make sure you mix hard workouts with easy ones, or days off) for muscle tissue recovery and building time. Remember, 50 percent of the building equation is rest; the other half is work! Don't use these approaches more than once or twice per week, and keep these tough workouts to no longer than 30 minutes and about 10 exercises. Perform one to two sets per exercise.

KEY POINT

After doing high-intensity strength training, take at least one day off before strength training again. After a day's rest, follow this type of workout with a strength workout that is of moderate or light intensity.

Following are several of the most highly used and effective high-intensity training techniques, many of which require a workout partner to assist. It's essential to have a spotter, for safety reasons, when using high-intensity strength training techniques.

BREAKDOWN TRAINING

This technique begins with a normal training set (i.e., 10 to 12 reps after a warm-up). Upon reaching momentary muscle failure, each exercise is performed with less weight than the one preceding it. Take off enough weight (usually about 10 to 20 percent) so that you can do two to four (more if you can) additional repetitions.

PYRAMID TRAINING

Pyramid training is a variation of breakdown training. Each exercise is performed with slightly less or more weight than the one preceding it. This results in you having an option of an up pyramid (weight increases) or a down pyramid (weight decreases). Let's say your goal is to start with a weight you can lift 10 to 12 times (10- to 12-RM). After fatiguing at 10- to 12-RM, you could take off about 10 to 20 percent of the weight (down pyramid) and force out more reps. Each time you reach a point at which you cannot complete any more reps, strip off additional weight, force more reps, and continue in this manner. Reversing the process creates an up pyramid, which is extremely difficult. In this situation, increasing the weight by as little as 5 percent is often sufficient, and you'll find that it is not too long before you cannot do even one repetition.

ASSISTED TRAINING OR FORCED REPS

Begin with a set of repetitions to fatigue (e.g., 10- to 12-RM). When you reach fatigue yet can still maintain good technique, your workout partner assists you in completing an additional number of reps you could not have completed on your own. Typically, the spotter lifts 10 to 15 percent of the weight load to assist you in completing two to four more reps (more if you can).

NEGATIVE TRAINING

Negative training allows for about 30 percent more muscle force production than concentric contraction. Typically, negative training is accomplished by (1) adding manual resistance on the lowering phase of any lift, (2) adjusting the weight lifted and lowered when using a selectorized plate machine—lighter when lifting and heavier when lowering, or (3) having your workout partner assist you through a concentric phase (lifting) with an amount of weight you could not lift on your own. Then, you lower the weight during the eccentric phase without the aid of the partner.

Like many of these high-intensity techniques, negative training is used with a highly trained individual who is plateaued with regard to strength gains. Although caution should be used with any of these techniques, delayed-onset muscle soreness is very common with this type of training, so it should not be used unless you are highly conditioned.

SUPER SLOW TRAINING

Slow training is often described as tedious, torturous, excruciating, and productive! Slow training takes the emphasis away from number of reps and weight being lifted and focuses on increasing the time of each repetition. Slower movement speed reduces any contribution from momentum toward completing the range of motion. This results in more tension on the muscle and total force development (meaning more muscle is used).

Super slow training is often referred to as 10-second training, although any number of seconds can be assigned to each lifting phase. A popular version is comprised of a 10-second concentric lifting phase, followed by a 5-second eccentric lowering phase for each repetition. You can also reverse the concentration by lifting in 5 seconds and following this with a 10-second eccentric emphasis. Aim for failure in about four to six reps. No miracle number of seconds will produce the best results. Record your results and experiment.

Super slow training repetitions can last from 15 to 60 seconds. However, if increases in strength and hypertrophy are your goal, keep the repetition length at about 15 seconds or less. As duration of the repetition is increased, the amount of weight that can be lifted decreases and each point of the range of motion receives less than an optimal strength stimulus. Remember, the key stimulus for strength overload is intensity, working harder for shorter durations.

SUPER SET TRAINING

Super setting can refer to working opposing muscle groups (paired agonist and antagonist muscles) in succession (e.g., biceps/triceps or chest/back). This is a common approach to training but allows for the muscle group(s) to recover while the opposing muscle group(s) is working.

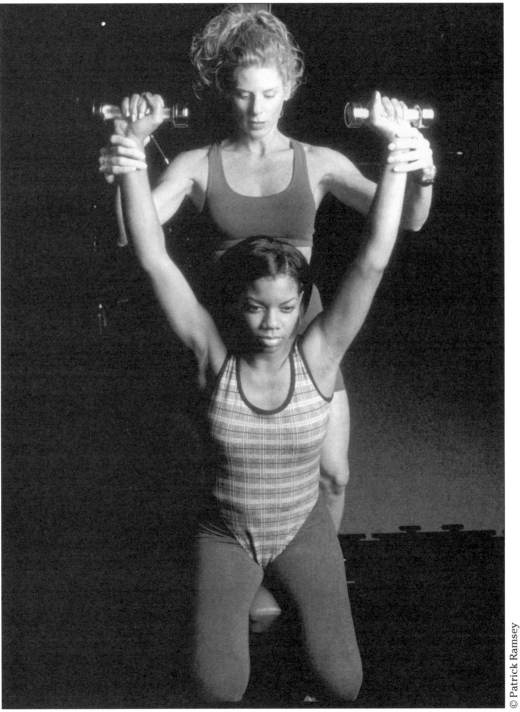

A partner can assist during the lifting (concentric) phase of negative training.

However, another type of super setting (sometimes referred to as compound training to distinguish the two) consists of working the same muscle group back to back—two sets of consecutive exercises target the same muscle group, but not necessarily with the same exercise. This type of super setting involves performing a set to fatigue, immediately followed by, or with little rest, additional sets and exercises that target the same muscle group. Super setting seems to work especially well in producing muscular hypertrophy when using a rep scheme of 6 to 10 repetitions to fatigue.

THE HIGH-INTENSITY TRAINING EDGE

If you've been training at an advanced level, high-intensity training may be the edge you need to move off strength plateaus. At some point in your advanced training program, if you're looking for more result within a limited time schedule, it's important to consider high-intensity strength training. High-volume work (working out more times per week and longer each workout) is not realistic in most personal schedules that require a balance between family, work, religion, health and fitness pursuits, and recreation. While high-volume work is somewhat effective with elite body builders and other professional athletes (remember, they do this for a living in many instances), it can lead to overuse injury and burnout. However, even when the time and motivation are present, many experts still argue that quality reigns over quantity when applied to training results. Many competitive lifters are experimenting with decreasing volume of overload and increasing intensity of effort.

> ### KEY POINT
> The best stimulus for increased gains in strength is to make the muscle work harder, not longer.

High-intensity strength training gives you a potential win-win situation. Use high-intensity training to maximize your result within a limited time schedule, but don't go overboard. Just as with volume training, science tells us that more is not always better, even if you have the time and desire! For optimal muscular development, variety and quality of training is the name of the game. Use periodization, which can encompass some or all of these techniques, as you vary your program on a regular basis (every three to four weeks).

Quick Index:

13 Peak to Compete

A balanced and effective team/individual anaerobic sport conditioning program will contain aerobic and anaerobic cardiovascular training, as well as strength, power (a combination of movement speed and strength), flexibility, quickness, agility, coordination, balance, and speed training. Likewise, the same is true for an effective team/individual endurance sport conditioning program. While one energy system (aerobic or anaerobic) may predominate during competition, both will need to be developed. It simply boils down to the degree of emphasis each area of training will receive.

Each approach to conditioning, whether it be for anaerobic team/individual sports or endurance team/individual sports, will require different adaptations in how often, how hard, and how long you work out. No single sport conditioning program can train you for a variety of activities that use different energy systems and movement patterns.

Nevertheless, when different kinds of workouts are needed within your training program, a simple approach that can help get your training on the right track is to identify the dominant type of training required of your particular sport or activity. For example, running a 10K race is dominated by aerobic metabolism, whereas tennis, downhill skiing, and ice hockey require short bursts of high-intensity or anaerobic effort. Once you've identified this aspect of the activity, use the following training programs to guide your workouts.

These programs will provide a safe and effective conditioning foundation with specific carryover to a variety of activities with different energy system demands. As your commitment to any individual sport moves beyond recreational or cross-training purposes, locate resources that detail in-depth, sport-specific training programs.

KEY POINT

No program is complete and effective at producing top performance unless it is balanced and specific. All aspects of fitness must be addressed in each training situation, even though a particular activity may be labeled as an anaerobic or aerobic activity.

TEAM AND INDIVIDUAL ANAEROBIC SPORTS

Many sports require up to 45 seconds of sustained, high-intensity effort followed by short rest periods or easy exercise. Sports such as tennis (skilled opponents playing a singles match typically rally for 5 to 10 seconds and hit 2 to 10 shots before a point is decided), volleyball (hard, sustained effort followed by recovery), basketball, and ice hockey (all-out efforts for about 45 seconds followed by rest) are good examples.

Stage one of any conditioning program is to get into shape. You may think that you're already fit, but are you (1) physically and mentally prepared for abrupt movement changes in upward, lateral, forward, and backward directions; (2) trained for quickness of movement and reaction time; (3) prepared to maintain short bursts of high-intensity effort over an entire match or game; (4) able to recover from bursts of anaerobic effort because you have a high level of aerobic conditioning; (5) flexible enough to provide the range of motion and pliability required of your body in the midst of demanding sport competition; and (6) capable of moving smoothly, effortlessly, and in control when performing at high intensity and speed (this represents coordination, balance, and agility)? By working on a sport conditioning circuit, you can turn any no answers into yes answers!

SPORT CONDITIONING CIRCUIT

A simple and effective way to train is to use a general sport conditioning circuit—a variety of fitness components with varying intensity organized to give you the best workout in the shortest time. This will provide you with a time-efficient way to train all of the fitness elements necessary for a well-rounded team/individual anaerobic sports conditioning workout. Plus, you will have added a very important element to any workout: FUN!

Your circuit can be laid out so that you progress from station to station, or it can be performed in unison. In other words, one small area, about four feet by eight feet, can be set aside for all of your equipment (e.g., adjustable step, lateral slide board, cones, tubing, mats, etc.). You set up as many stations as you can in this small area and rearrange stations as necessary as you go through the circuit. (One of the tricks of a well-balanced circuit is to use equipment suggested in the section on equipment because of if its versatility; it can be used for more than one station.)

Additionally, you may choose to perform only five to six of the suggested stations (I've created a 16-station sport conditioning circuit for you), and you can add exercises that you come up with. You can get ideas for additional stations from conditioning drills you've participated in during sport clinics or use lessons learned from a golf or tennis pro or other professional coach. The sky is the limit with regard to station options, but above all else, train hard and have fun!

Sport Conditioning Equipment

To make this circuit more fun, interesting, and effective, you should have the ultimate bag of toys. However, this equipment is not necessary to create an effective and fun circuit. Use your imagination and creativeness to create the circuit if you have limited equipment options. For example, do you really need a jump rope to "phantom" or "air" jump? Paper cups, chalk, or duct tape can be used in place of cones.

The following is a list of useful equipment options:

- Chronograph, stopwatch, whistle
- Stability balls (air-filled balls used especially for abdominal and back work)
- Weighted balls (you toss these back and forth with a training partner or hold them, for example, when performing crunches to add more weight)
- Step platforms and slide boards
- Plyometric jump boxes
- Elastic resistance (tubing)
- Balance board, mats, minitramps (help develop balance and coordination—just try standing on one and you'll feel the balance challenge)
- Pylon cones, colored tape, chalk (create your agility and speed patterns on the floor)
- Jump ropes
- Assorted balls (basketball, soccer, etc.)
- Your imagination!

Sport Conditioning Circuit Overview

This circuit emphasizes anaerobic conditioning (cardiovascular and strength) and agility movement patterns to complement activities such as tennis, volleyball, and ice hockey. Anaerobic cardiovascular stations (anaerobic and aerobic intervals challenge the short-term lactic acid energy system) and anaerobic strength stations (about 6 to 15 controlled repetitions to fatigue or 12 to 15 if you don't have progressive overload equipment—such as tubes and weights—available) both last 30 to 90 seconds.

Aerobic stations (don't confuse this with aerobic interval training) can be inserted into this circuit and should last about three to four minutes. Aerobic training is steady-rate training. You would classify this level of effort as easy to maintain for durations longer than three to five minutes. Aerobic training helps your body recover quickly from hard anaerobic effort. This includes strength and interval training. Aerobic efforts should be "moderate" to "somewhat hard," versus "hard," to "very hard" for anaerobic cardiovascular efforts. Thus, both types of training can be used in this program. One type of training is not exclusive of the other! If you're an anaerobic athlete and don't have a good base of aerobic conditioning, add five or six of these longer-duration stations to your circuit.

The circuit may be performed once or repeated several times. Fit it into your training schedule based on your goals and planned training session. Additionally, it can be used once or twice per week or less frequently depending on your training needs.

Sport Conditioning Circuit: Station by Station

Warm up for at least three to five minutes before beginning the circuit, and be sure to conclude with a cool-down (three to five minutes) and stretching.

Station 1: Jumping Rope

Use a variety of foot and arm patterns that include two-feet landings, one-foot jumping, arm crossovers, and side-to-side jumping. If you don't want to actually jump over the rope as it crosses under your feet, phantom jump. Simply twirl the rope side to side in front of your body as you jump. The duration should be between 30 and 90 seconds.

Station 2: Lateral Hop

Perform the lateral hops quickly (move as though your feet are touching hot coals) and in a direction that travels laterally and forward at the same time (this is not the same as hopping side to side, which can cause unnecessary stress to the knee). You can create any pattern of movement that mimics the activity patterns you are training to improve. The duration should be between 30 and 90 seconds.

Station 3: Lateral Sliding

If you don't own a slideboard, substitute shuffling laterally. Your lateral training board should have end ramps that are slightly angled (like a ramp) and turned out. After you push off, maintain a low-profile position (athletic ready) and keep your feet wide until your lead foot contacts the other ramp. The total duration should be between 30 and 90 seconds.

Station 4: Athletic Stepping

Perform basic or propulsion (step up and propel yourself upward, landing on the step/platform) step movements on a step that can be adjusted from four to eight inches. Athletic stepping prepares your body for impact and eccentric muscle contractions (downhill skiing is a great example) that commonly occur in sport movements. Never jump from the step to the floor. Instead, step up onto

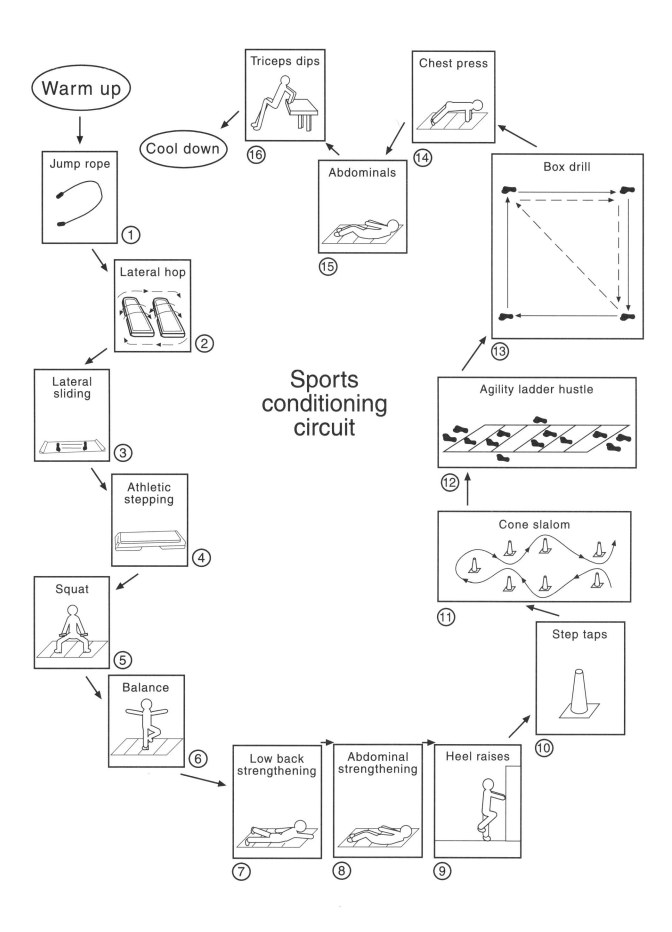

Warm up

Jump rope ①

Lateral hop ②

Lateral sliding ③

Athletic stepping ④

Squat ⑤

Balance ⑥

Cool down

Triceps dips ⑯

Abdominals ⑮

Chest press ⑭

Box drill ⑬

Agility ladder hustle ⑫

Cone slalom ⑪

Step taps ⑩

Low back strengthening ⑦

Abdominal strengthening ⑧

Heel raises ⑨

Sports conditioning circuit

the platform as you face it, propel yourself upward by taking off from one foot, and land on the elevated step platform. Then, step off. The duration should be between 30 and 90 seconds.

You can also do a propulsion version called "across-the-top." Stand to the side of the platform at either end, facing forward. With the foot closest to the step, step to the middle of the platform, take off from this leg and as you move sideways, the other (outside) leg sets down on top of the platform as the lead leg (inside) contacts the floor on the opposite side of the platform.

Station 5: Squat

Use tubing or dumbbells to perform this strength exercise with adequate resistance. The duration should be between 30 and 90 seconds (6 to 12 six-second reps to fatigue).

Station 6: Balance

Balance training can be as simple as standing on one leg on an unstable surface such as an exercise mat. The goal is to train the stabilizing muscles of the ankle, knee, and hip. If you have access to, or own, a balance board, this piece of equipment offers additional balance challenges. You should attempt a duration of 30 seconds with each leg.

Station 7: Low Back Strengthening

Lie face down and simultaneously reach out with your right arm and lift your left leg. After you tire, repeat on the other side. For a tougher challenge, perform a back extension by lying face down. Place your hands at your sides or under your chin (harder) and raise your chest off the ground with control. Add a subtle rotation after you've mastered the back extension. If you own a stability ball, you can perform these same exercises on the ball. The ball adds an additional stability challenge (follow the manual or video that should accompany this piece of equipment). The duration should be between 30 and 90 seconds to muscle fatigue (12 to 15 controlled reps).

Station 8: Abdominal Strengthening

Lie on your back and perform traditional ab work, reverse hip lifts or curls, and abdominal isolation with rotation. If you own a stability ball, you can perform these same exercises on the ball. The ball adds an additional stability challenge (follow the manual or video that should accompany this piece of equipment). The duration should be between 30 and 90 seconds to muscle fatigue (12 to 15 controlled reps).

Station 9: Unilateral Heel Raise

Stand with your feet about 12 inches from a wall. Place your right foot so that it is in line with the center of your body. Place the left foot behind the right lower leg and above the ankle. Rise up on the ball of the foot until tired and repeat on the other leg. The duration should be between 30 and 90 seconds (12 to 15 controlled reps).

Station 10: Step Taps

Stand in front of a cone or step (about eight inches high). Alternately (and quickly) jump from foot to foot. As you land on one foot, extend the other leg outward and lightly tap the top of the cone or step platform. Keep your chest upright and your shoulders aligned over your hips. The duration should be between 30 and 90 seconds.

Station 11: Cone Slalom

Dribble a ball in a slalom fashion around a series of cones. Include several directional changes that involve forward, backward, and lateral (sideways) slalom dribbling. The duration should be between 30 and 90 seconds.

Station 12: Agility Ladder Hustle

Use tape or chalk (commercial agility ladders made of nylon strapping and dowel ladder rungs are available) to create your ladder. This is not unlike hopscotch, in that your goal is to create various foot patterns. Try to move quickly, lightly, and accurately through your course. The duration should be between 30 and 90 seconds.

Station 13: Box Drill

Create a box perimeter of any size (eight feet by eight feet is a great size, but smaller is OK) with cones, chalk, or tape. Stay inside the perimeter and mix shuffle steps in box, star, triangle, and side-to-side patterns. Use directional changes (go the other way) liberally and change the direction your body faces with quarter, half, and full pivots. The duration should be between 30 and 90 seconds.

Station 14: Chest Press

Perform a traditional push-up (or modified—your knees are in contact with the mat). If you have a bench and dumbbells or tubing available and your goal is to optimize strength gains, select the resistance that will fatigue you in 6 to 12 reps. If you own a stability ball, you can perform these exercises on the ball. The ball adds an additional stability challenge (follow the manual or video that should accompany this piece of equipment). The duration should be between 30 and 90 seconds (12 to 15 reps with control).

Station 15: Abdominal Strengthening

Follow the directions for station 8 (this is to provide recovery time for upper body exercises).

Station 16: Triceps Dips

Use a step platform or bench to raise you from the ground. Place your hands securely over the edge of the bench nearest you and just wider than your shoulders. Keep your back in contact with the bench or step as you slowly lower your body. Maintain control and don't allow your upper arms to go lower than parallel to the ground. The duration should be between 30 and 90 seconds (12 to 15 reps with control).

KEY POINT

Remember to cool down and stretch once you've finished your workout!

ENDURANCE SPORT TRAINING

Regardless of your endurance sport (running, walking, triathlon, cycling, swimming, etc.), a balanced approach is necessary. Cardiovascular conditioning, which should include interval training, is the hallmark of your program. Nevertheless, the right kind of strength training will help you whether you're getting your aerobic workout in the water, in a group exercise step class, cycling on the road, or scrambling (running, hiking, walking, or mountain biking) on trails.

Following is an endurance sport progression that you can use for any endurance sport that lasts from 15 minutes to an hour and beyond. I've created this workout using duration (minutes) rather than specific distances so that it will be applicable to all endurance sports. Don't forget to add stretching and strength training to form a balanced approach to endurance sport training.

Is your goal simply to finish a 5K, 10K, or marathon event? Or are you trying to win the race or go your fastest? Maybe your interest is road cycling, mountain biking, swimming, cross-country skiing (striding or skate skiing), race or fitness walking, or running. As different as these events are with regard to skill practice and acquisition, their common trait is that the heart muscle must be strong and able to deliver large quantities of oxygen efficiently so you can endure over long periods of time. Additionally, the muscles must be trained (specificity of training) and able to use the oxygen (oxygen extraction) that passes by them via the blood. And, each of these sports represents an activity that could be described as rhythmical, uses large muscle groups, and generally is sustained longer than several minutes. That's why a progressive endurance program based on duration can work equally well for any of these endurance sports.

Endurance Sport Training Program

Any type of training program is enhanced when you have an aerobic training base. The first phase of any endurance program is to lay the aerobic foundation and to maintain it through the year. If you have been training progressively (30 minutes three or four times per week for four to six weeks), you can skip basic training and move on to building your endurance program.

> **KEY POINT**
>
> Remember, any aerobic-based activity can be used in this program. Don't limit yourself to the examples. Simply place the aerobic activity of your choice into the following training schedule; it works!

To gauge your intensity, you will be given perceived exertion levels (RPE) to attain. The 1 to 10 RPE scale (or effort scale) is explained in chapter 5.

Foundation Training (Basic Training)

Goal:	To run 2–3 miles (enter a 5K/3.1-mile race), or cycle or swim 15–20 minutes continuously
Frequency:	2–3 times per week
Intensity (RPE):	2–3 ("somewhat easy" to "moderate")
Time:	10–15 minutes (done continuously or in separate, for example, 10-minute and 5-minute, segments)
Length of stage:	2–3 weeks

Description: Exercising continuously for 15 to 20 minutes requires a manageable starting point. You could start with a walk/run or easy bike ride outdoors for 10 minutes and ride indoors on a stationary cycle for 5 minutes for a total of 15 minutes. You get the idea. Training consistently for a few weeks will prepare your body for additional minutes of training and a new level of endurance fitness. While you're building your base, it's OK to stick with one activity, or if you have another favorite, cross-train.

Building Your Endurance Program

Stage I goal:	To run, bike, or swim for increasing durations; maybe complete a 5K (3.1-mile) race or a 15-mile bike ride
Frequency:	3 times per week
Intensity (RPE):	3–4 ("moderate" to "somewhat hard")
Time:	20–30 minutes
Length of stage:	2–3 weeks

Description: Increase duration gradually (never more than 10 percent of current duration) and allow two to three weeks to stabilize. This level of effort should feel easy with no discomfort before you advance to stage II. To complete a 5K (3.1-mile) race or bike strongly for 30 minutes, you need to train at least three times per week at an RPE of 3 to 4 for 20 to 30 minutes. Don't forget to cross-train and mix in easy aerobic efforts.

Stage II goal:	To move beyond a strong aerobic base of fitness; maybe run a 10K (6.2-mile) race or complete a 25-mile bike ride
Frequency:	3–5 times per week
Intensity (RPE):	3–5 ("moderate" to "somewhat hard")
Time:	30–40 minutes
Length of stage:	3–4 weeks

Description: If your easy running pace is an eight-minute mile, one long run of 40 minutes per week should prepare you and make you feel confident enough to complete a 10K. Don't forget to cross-train and mix in easy aerobic efforts.

Advanced Endurance Training

Stage I goal: Long duration efforts; to become a long-distance athlete

Frequency: 4–6 times per week

Intensity (RPE):   3–6 ("moderate" to "hard")

Time: 40–60 minutes

Length of stage: 4–6 weeks

Description: Progression, patience, and consistency are the keys. Pay special attention to overtraining signals (pain, fatigue, exhaustion that doesn't go away after workouts) and listen carefully to how your body is responding to this high volume of cardiovascular training. Don't forget to cross-train and mix in easy aerobic efforts. Take a day off when you feel burned out. This is a lot of exercise!

Stage II goal: To introduce high-intensity anaerobic interval training and aerobic interval training; to optimize cardiovascular fitness

Frequency: Once or twice per week

Intensity (RPE):   4–7 ("somewhat hard" to "very hard") for aerobic intervals; 7–9 ("very hard" to "very, very hard") for anaerobic intervals

Time: 1.5–3.0 minutes for aerobic intervals; 30–90 seconds for anaerobic intervals

Length of stage: After your base of conditioning is developed, use regularly throughout your training

Description: Interval training, along with aerobic or steady-rate ("easy" to "moderate") training, allows you to fully develop your cardiovascular system. Don't forget to cross-train and mix in easy aerobic efforts of short and longer durations.

Strength Training for the Endurance Athlete

Typically, competitive endurance athletes allocate only about 10 to 15 percent of their total training time to a strength program. If the athlete is nearing the start of the competition season, this may decrease to 5 percent. Carefully evaluate whether you're looking for elite endurance performance or whether you'd like to see great results in both strength and cardiovascular endurance. Thirty percent, or more, of your program may be allotted to strength training if you're looking for significant fitness gains in both areas.

Even athletes who specialize in endurance should prioritize strength training for at least three months of their training year. This helps prepare them for the competitive season, and their strength gains can easily be maintained by training only twice per week.

Endurance athletes looking for top performance do not need excessive muscle mass (especially for running or other activities in which you have to carry extra body weight!). However, they need to be strong to protect their joints and back, maintain correct form and posture, and gain a performance advantage.

You can gain significant strength without simultaneously building huge muscles. Your muscles can become stronger through neural adaptations (you

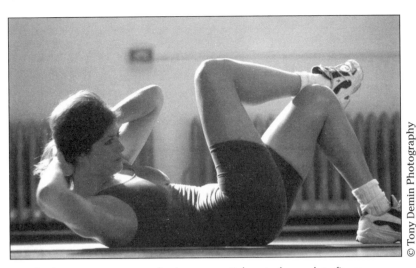

Developing strong core muscles is an essential part of complete fitness.

can recruit muscle fibers that were "sleeping" or not being used) and by increasing muscle size (you can minimize hypertrophy by using a slightly higher rep scheme of 12 to 15 or 15 to 20 reps to fatigue). Strength training can enhance muscle endurance and power, prevent injury, delay fatigue, and give you a psychological advantage. You will feel strong!

Follow phases I and II of the strength periodization program in chapter 11 to build your strength base. Progress through phases III and IV to peak your strength and power gains. Finish Phase IV six to eight weeks before your competitive season starts, and maintain your strength and power gains by training 12 to 15 reps to fatigue for each exercise and by performing one or two sets twice per week.

KEY POINT

If you're specializing as an endurance athlete, you can keep your strength training to a minimum and still get the results you need by training smart!

As you design your training approach, chapters 2 through 8 can help you with the nuts and bolts of cardiovascular, strength, and flexibility training, as well as show you how to organize and progress your program. Regardless of your training goal, program design is nothing more than varied combinations of how often (frequency), how long (duration), and how hard (intensity) you train. As you create conditioning programs for different goals, you will notice considerable overlap, which should make your program design challenges even easier. Balanced and effective programming will always require that all of the major components of fitness be challenged.

Quick Index:

14 Design Your Own Program

Versatile and effective program design requires an optimal combination of activities that specifically meet your health and fitness needs and changing fitness levels. This is purposeful training (as opposed to a random selection of activities) based on goals, benefits, and activity preferences.

Your Personal Trainer gives you the tools to develop a workout plan that uses a variety of activities and keeps you progressing. Your activities and program emphasis can change from workout to workout, week to week, or month to month when you use the concepts of cross-training and periodization.

The combination of activities chosen and the intensity and the percentage of time per workout given each activity will be based on specific goals. Using scientific principles of periodization (varying intensity, duration, and frequency over time), you will be able to create (or follow in this book) different workouts that can be cycled in three- or four-week time periods. This can help you stay interested, help you stick with your training, and optimize your training results. *Your Personal Trainer* will help you attain your goals more quickly than you would using a random selection of activities and an unplanned approach to training.

DETERMINING YOUR GOALS

Remember to choose goals that are appropriate, realistic, and of interest to you. If you're not motivated and excited about your new goals, they won't be accomplished. The following are some goal categories for you to consider.

Goal Categories

Some of your goals may already be incorporated into your training program. Others might spur you to conclude that your approach was not as comprehensive and balanced as it could be. Be sure to choose a variety of long- and short-term goals and plan your workouts accordingly. And remember, you can emphasize one goal over another, but probably not all of the time. (For example, you may want to periodize your program and emphasize strength training for about eight weeks using 80 percent of your allotted exercise time to attain new levels of strength.)

Weight Loss, Weight Management, and Fat Burning

This category emphasizes equal amounts of cardiovascular activity (for calorie and fat burning) and strength training (to build lean mass and increase metabolic rate). The ratio should be 50 percent cardiovascular activities (don't forget to include some interval training) and 50 percent strength activities.

Improving Cardiovascular Fitness

This category emphasizes steady-rate (easy, cruising effort) aerobic activities and interval training (harder work efforts). The ratio should be 60 percent aerobic cardiovascular activities, 20 percent anaerobic cardiovascular activities (interval training), and 20 percent strength activities (focusing on trunk stability—abs, back, and upper body).

Improving Muscle Strength and Endurance

This category emphasizes strength training to improve muscle tone, sculpt or define the body, and improve strength. The ratio should be 80 percent strength activities and 20 percent aerobic activities.

Improving Overall Health

This category emphasizes balance among the three components of fitness to reduce stress, improve flexibility, reduce the risks of heart disease and orthopedic problems, and slow the aging process. The ratio should be 35 percent aerobic activities, 35 percent strength activities, and 30 percent flexibility activities.

Sample Workout

Most of your workouts will take from 30 minutes to an hour and a half to complete. You can fit your workout into any time format. The given activity ratios are for the actual workout portion of the session. Remember to subtract your warm-up and cool-down times from the total duration and then figure the activity times for each fitness component with the remaining time.

There are an infinite number of exercise choices you can use to keep your interest level high and meet your fitness goals. Activities can be sequenced in numerous ways. For example, individual activities within a component of fitness can be varied from workout to workout if you want more variety. Or, the same activities can be repeated in each workout using a different sequence. Make sure you select activities that fall into the three important components of fitness, which include cardiovascular, strength, and stretching activities.

Short-term goals can be changed (updated) at the end of any three- or four-week cycle, and a new program created to meet the new standard at which you're aiming. It's a good idea to focus on consistent training for a minimum of three weeks in order to derive benefits from that training.

Example

Total workout time:	60 minutes
Goal:	Weight loss, weight management, and fat burning
Warm-up:	5 minutes
Cool-down/stretch:	7 minutes
Activities:	Cardiovascular activities—24 minutes (50%)
	(i.e., 8 minutes stationary cycling, 8 minutes running on a treadmill, 8 minutes stair stepping, or 24 minutes walking outside)
	Strength activities—24 minutes (50%)
	(i.e., 8 minutes free weights, 8 minutes tubing, 8 minutes machine, or 24 minutes using only dumbbells or free weights)

TEN STEPS TO PROGRAM DESIGN

Take the time to plan and periodize your program. One-size-fits-all program design does not work. As you probably already know, you have unique needs, interests, and responses to various activities and training protocols. Because of this, you need to put some forethought into your training program. Do this before you jump into an unplanned mess. Not only will this frustrate you, but you won't get the results you want and you might even quit!

> ### KEY POINT
>
> If your workout is retelling the same old story day in and day out, you will not progress. Working out must go beyond a well-intentioned flurry of unplanned activity.

By moving through each of these 10 steps, you have a format that ensures your training is built on a solid foundation of science while being customized to your individual needs.

Step 1: Information Gathering

The information-gathering process involves two steps: (1) completing a health history questionnaire and (2) self-testing your fitness level (optional).

The medical history/health questionnaire asks questions that elicit information you need to help identify medical concerns, your personal understanding of basic fitness concepts, current and past fitness activities, goals and interests, and eating habits.

Fitness self-testing is an *optional* motivational tool that you can use to define a starting point and motivate yourself to change your fitness program over time. In no way should it be used as a diagnostic tool that assesses whether you have an illness or not. Fitness testing *can* be highly motivational to certain individuals.

Typically, personal trainers test submaximal cardiovascular fitness, muscle strength and endurance, flexibility, and body composition (percent body fat). The results serve as a benchmark from which further improvements can be objectively measured. To do so, the exact procedure used in the initial test must be replicated in the retest. For example, a positive adaptation to cardiovascular training could be a lower heart rate for a given work load (the level of effort you worked at on the previous test). Heart rate is an example of a tangible and objective measure of improvement—or lack of improvement—in fitness over a specific time period. For any test to be a valid measure of your progress, you must repeat the exact testing procedure each time.

Step 2: Balanced Physical Programming

Balanced physical programming includes cardiovascular conditioning, muscular strength and endurance conditioning, and flexibility training. All of these key components of fitness must be addressed correctly to ensure that you have taken a balanced approach to your health and fitness.

Within each component, you likewise balance fitness. For example, within the muscular strength and endurance component, all agonist and antagonist muscle pairs, such as the biceps and triceps, need to be challenged.

Balanced physical programming walks a fine line between listening to what you want and incorporating these interests into a program that also contains what you *need* from a total wellness perspective. Don't neglect to understand the importance of including all the components.

Step 3: Cardiovascular Conditioning

Cardiovascular conditioning is activity that involves large-muscle, rhythmic, continuous movement that simultaneously increases heart rate and blood flow back to the heart. This type of conditioning can decrease the risk factors associated with heart disease, increase endurance and personal vitality, and help with weight maintenance or loss. Use a variety of cardio activities (walking, running, biking, swimming) to challenge the heart and lungs and to avoid the increased risk of overuse injury associated with unrelenting and repetitive motions.

Step 4: Muscular Strength and Endurance Conditioning

Most people should engage in strength training. Proper strength training can boost metabolism, increase lean muscle, help decrease fat mass or maintain ideal weight, decrease the risk for osteoporosis, increase self-esteem, preserve personal physical independence, and increase strength.

Effective muscular strength and endurance conditioning is dependent on a progressive increase in resistance over time that challenges all of the major muscles. Be sure to train all of the body's paired agonist/antagonist (or opposing) muscle groups.

Step 5: Flexibility Training

Healthy, or desired, flexibility is a capacity to move freely in every intended direction. Adapting the concept of functional range of motion (FROM) and using active range of motion (AROM) technique in your flexibility programming may allow you to participate more effectively in daily domestic activities and recreational pursuits with less potential for injury. Since flexibility is specific to each joint's musculature, design a program that stretches areas of the body that are often lacking in adequate flexibility and target all major muscles since flexibility is joint specific (you may be mobile in one joint and tight in another).

Step 6: Active Rest

Regardless of your fitness level, thread the concept of active rest throughout your fitness routines. The active rest concept sequences exercises to structure a workout that optimizes workout time and accommodates your fitness level. Typically, a large amount of time in traditional fitness programs involves recovery from work performed. Following are several ways to minimize wasted recovery time or to eliminate it.

1. Use perceived exertion and intervals (work, recovery) to keep you moving continuously during cardiovascular conditioning.
2. Sequence resistance training exercises so that they alternate from muscle group to muscle group, or from upper to lower body to abs and back exercises.
3. If a muscle group is targeted for consecutive multiple sets, the recovery phase(s) can be used for flexibility training.

If you're looking for maximum results with minimum time investment, active rest is an excellent way to optimize the finite time you have available.

Step 7: Cross-Training

Cross-training is fun! Its use in your program leads to productive and time-efficient activity that helps you achieve your goals.

You can cross-train within a component of fitness, such as cardiovascular fitness (running, walking, stepping, etc.), or between components of fitness (use a circuit with muscular endurance and cardiovascular fitness emphasized). Using cross-training within your program gives you big advantages, such as

- variety and change,
- new physiological stimulation (new fitness gains), and
- the motivation to stick with it.

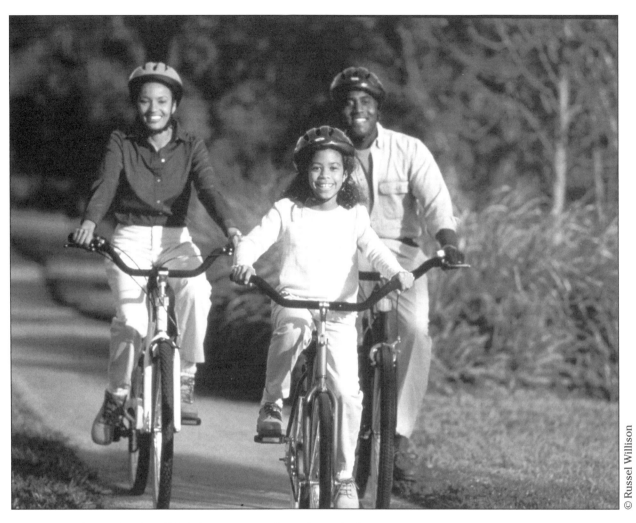

Exercising with your family will help keep your workouts fun and relaxing.

Some people like change and some do not. Changing for the sake of variety is the wrong reason. Change is best implemented when you're ready physiologically (your body is hurting and/or not responding) and psychologically (your mind is suffering and training is no longer fun).

Step 8: Awareness of Special Needs

Everyone has special concerns. You already have the tools to balance fitness among cardiovascular, muscular strength and endurance, and flexibility components. Now you will need to consider issues such as exercise for performance versus fitness versus health, safe weight maintenance and loss, strength plateaus, or pregnancy. You may also need to address nutritional concerns or motivational and psychological needs. You will need to determine what kind of self-talk (yes, you need to have a chat now and then with yourself) will keep you exercising. Taking all of these things into account will help you design the perfect customized program.

Step 9: Success and Adherence

Feeling that you are successful is one—if not the most—important aspect of program design. Four factors ensure exercise adherence and a successful program.

1. Time—keep most workouts to around one hour two to four times per week. If you have special training needs, go for it and train more!
2. Variety—use cross-training when appropriate and periodize your program.
3. Intrinsic motivation—you should know *why* you want to exercise (ask yourself!).
4. Lifestyle changes—you must like what you are doing to incorporate a training approach or other new behavior into a lifelong routine.

Step 10: The Reality Factor

No individual is the perfect model of textbook programming. The key to focus on is the degree of your individual improvement. Is your life better? Have you accomplished short-term goals on a regular basis? Rather than create a program that a fitness professional would approve of, attempt to optimize your involvement in fitness for a lifetime, with whatever techniques it takes.

Don't be a robotic exerciser who uses one recipe/program all the time. Fitness programming is not a clear-cut issue. More often than not, an effective program is composed of a smorgasbord of options that shift in concert with your ever-changing needs. *Your Personal Trainer* provides the buffet table (low-fat, of course!) from which to choose.

Quick Index:

PART IV

Your Training Targets

15 Track Your Progress

John Wooden, the legendary UCLA basketball coach, said, "Don't let what you cannot do interfere with what you can do." It's too easy to get bogged down with what you have not accomplished (that's what long-term goals are for!). Focus on the positive, what you can do and have done, and applaud how far you have come from where you started.

In chapter 1 we discussed the importance of knowing where you've been, where you are, and where you'd like to go in order to create a goal- and results-oriented training program. In the earlier chapters of this book, you recorded a starting point from which to compare your fitness improvements over time—but remember, it was only a starting point. You need to keep track of your progress continually by reassessing your fitness level periodically. Results reflect what you are achieving and doing—not what you think you are doing.

REASSESSING YOUR FITNESS LEVEL

Ongoing reassessment is essential if you are to objectively measure your progress, or lack thereof. This regular checkup of your fitness program is important to hold you accountable for making changes that are needed and for giving you a pat on the back for a job well done! Tracking and evaluating your progress will help you achieve your goals and keep your workouts focused and on target.

When to Test and Retest

While you are encouraged to test yourself when starting your program, you may want to create a foundation of conditioning first. Regardless of when you first self-test, retesting six to eight weeks after the initial tests makes sense because you'll likely see great improvements if you're working out regularly, eating right, and following the guidelines in this book. These significant before and after improvements will serve to further motivate you. Testing again at six months, one year, and at least once a year thereafter is a reasonable plan to follow. If you want to test more frequently, feel free to do so.

Tracking Your Progress

The results of your tests may be recorded on the various recording/testing sheets located in chapter 1. Keeping track of your results is important so that you can see how much you improve from test date to test date. These self-tests will also tell you whether your exercise programs and eating plan are working.

Unfortunately, most test results are filed away to collect dust. Don't let this happen! Your results can show you the areas of fitness that you need to improve in and simultaneously motivate you to keep progressing. If you're new to training, you'll probably see outstanding improvement during the first three months of training. After this time period, results will come at a less dramatic pace, but steadily. Understanding this fact about training improvements will keep you—whether a veteran or a beginning exerciser—from developing unrealistic expectations.

KEY POINT

Self-testing is not only a smart approach toward optimizing training results, but also highly motivating.

Using Performance Graphs

Performance graphs are an excellent tool to use if you want to get an overall picture of the direction your training is headed. Over a period of weeks, these graphs should also show increased results for three to four weeks, followed by a plateau or dip, followed by another three- to four-week increase period. This rise, followed by a leveling or slight dip, reflects a properly periodized program which allows for both hard training and recovery.

The performance graph has both a vertical and a horizontal axis or line. The vertical line represents your performance, as measured by past and most current (1) body fat measurements (as you get more fit, your body fat will go down, so a positive graph for this test will start high and go down!), (2) strength self-tests, (3) cardiovascular self-tests (as you get more fit, your heart rate will go down, so a positive graph for this test will, again, start high and go down!), and (4) amount of weight being lifted for a particular strength exercise. One of my clients' favorite results to record on the performance graph is personal percentage improvement, which you will learn how to calculate later in this chapter. These few examples demonstrate how easy it is to end up with a bar graph or performance line for almost any fitness-related task.

The horizontal line of the performance graph represents time. Generally, it is easiest to record improvement by weeks and months.

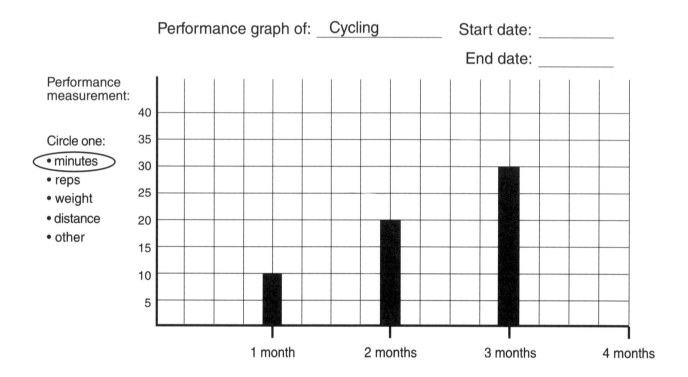

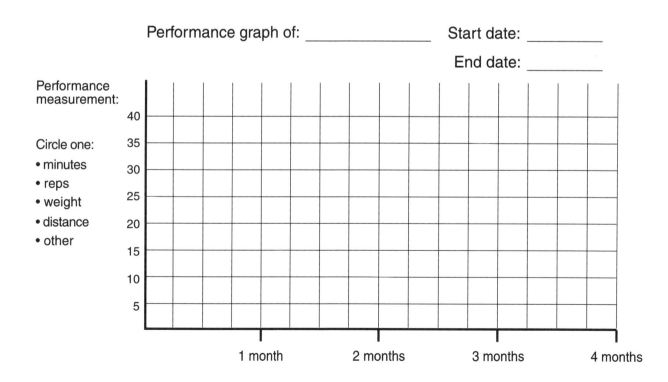

WEEK-AT-A-GLANCE WORKOUT LOG

Let's say you have detailed and recorded your workouts for a period of time (about six months to a year) using the various record-keeping and goal-setting sheets provided in chapter 2. You might reach a point at which you want to further streamline your record-keeping process. Week-at-a-Glance will keep you in touch and accountable for your workout planning and journaling of your workout efforts, but it is even quicker. It takes you only a few minutes to enter your goals(s), resting pulse, type of workout, distances, intensities, and overall comments as to your general feeling about the workout. Do not completely stop

Sample Week-at-a-Glance Workout Log					
Goal	Day	AM pulse	Workout description	Cardio* distance/time	Comments
Moderate cardio workout	Mon	60	Easy run, light stretching after the run, abdominal and back strength exercises	50 minutes	Starting to feel tired; needed an easy workout
Full body strength workout	Tue	65	6–8 reps today, per set, target all of the muscle groups	35 minutes	Cut my workout short; body feels heavy
Interval workout	Wed	68	Canceled workout; just not feeling good	N/A	I need a rest!
Light stationary bike and strength workout	Thu	62	45 minutes on bike; some easy speed play; full body strength workout using 12–15 reps to fatigue	45 minutes on bike plus 30 minutes strength time	Rest felt great; body's starting to respond again; training is fun! Glad I changed my workout plans.
Rest	Fri	62	Complete rest/recovery	N/A	Feeling good, but I want to keep in my planned rest day.
Long run	Sat	59	90-minute run with easy intervals (20-second pickups followed by easy recovery); 20-minute stretch	90 minutes plus stretch time	Stretch felt great, needed that! Back on track, run felt easy and comfortable.
Family time	Sun	61	2–3 hour hike with light pack, moderate pace	about 3 hours	Nice!! Will do 3 hard strength workouts next week.

* Detail your strength workout on the record-keeping sheet found in chapter 11 called Week-at-a-Glance Strength Workout Sheet.

			Week-at-a-Glance Workout Log		
Goal	Day	AM Pulse	Workout Description	Cardio* Distance/Time	Comments
	Mon				
	Tue				
	Wed				
	Thu				
	Fri				
	Sat				
	Sun				

*Detail your strength workout on the record-keeping sheet found in chapter 11 called Week-at-a-Glance Strength Workout Sheet.

using the in-depth planning/recording sheets you initially used. It might be important to revisit them periodically to keep you on track. If you prefer the forms in chapter 2, keep using them!

CALCULATING YOUR PERCENT IMPROVEMENT

Fitness assessment and testing results can be used for (1) comparing your test results to the results of others who have taken the test and (2) calculating your personal percent improvement.

Calculate Percent Improvement

Fitness component	(a) Initial or previous test result	(b) Retest #1 or most recent test result	(c) Difference between previous and most recent test result (a − b)	(d) Difference divided by initial or previous test result [(c ÷ a) × 100]
Cardiovascular (heart rate in beats/minute)	168 beats/minute	142 beats/minute	26 beats/minute	26 ÷ 168 = .1547; .1547 × 100 = about 16% improvement
Strength (repetitions completed)	8 repetitions	13 repetitions	5 repetitions	5 ÷ 8 = .625; .625 × 100 = about 63% improvement
Cardiovascular (time for one-mile walk test)	28 minutes	20 minutes	8 minutes	8 ÷ 28 = .286 .286 × 100 = about 29% improvement

By comparing your test results to the scores (norms or percentiles) of other people who have taken the tests, you are able to rate your effort using terms such as *excellent, average,* and *poor.* Norm comparisons also let you see how you compare to other people of your age and gender. Or, you may be placed in a percentile ranking. For example, if you're at the 90th percentile, you have performed better than 90 percent of the people who have taken this test. On the other hand, if you are rated at the 10th percentile, 90 percent of the people who have taken the test have done better than you.

I often call this the judgment scale. Norms are a double-edged sword that can motivate or demotivate, depending on how the scale rates your performance. In my opinion, any improvement, regardless of the starting point, is positive. Norm ratings may still leave you in the lowest category, even after great improvement.

The second method, personal percent improvement, compares your assessment results only to your starting point and subsequent tests. For many people it is more useful and motivating to show fitness changes that relate to their starting points. You may find it very disheartening to be compared to a standard of excellence (norms or percentiles) that seems impossible to achieve at this time in your health and fitness journey. It doesn't matter where you start, as long as you improve!

Percent improvement for *any* test is easily calculated by subtracting the most recent test result from that of the previous test. This difference is then divided by the previous test result and multiplied by 100. For the percentage improvement to reflect accurately your improvements (validity) related to previous efforts, the retest must be set up exactly the same way (just follow the procedures in chapter 1).

The following example shows how to calculate percent improvement for an individual's previous and most recent cardiovascular (based on heart rate recorded), strength (based on number of repetitions completed), and cardiovascular (based on number of minutes walked) self-assessment tests.

Improvement in fitness is reflected by heart rate and walking time *decreasing* and number of repetitions *increasing*. The newest testing results are compared to the previous or initial test. Based on this example, improvements of about 16, 63, and 29 percent are documented. Now, that's motivating! Who knows where norms or percentile rankings would leave you. I encourage you to graph your percentage improvement results on the reproducible performance graph on page 236.

HOW TO MAINTAIN YOUR FITNESS GAINS

What happens if you travel, get sick, or need some time off because you're overtrained? If you take a few days of planned rest, are your training results going to spiral down the drain? What is the most efficient way to keep fit? Is there a way to maintain your gains in fitness when you don't have the time to work out the way you'd like to?

Everyone wants to know how easily they can lose, or regain, their hard-won training benefits. It is true that you can't store exercise, and detraining (starting to lose your fitness benefits) starts to occur fairly rapidly once you stop exercising.

The positive side is that fitness gains may not be lost as quickly as you might think. Additional good news is that it may take *less* exercise than you think to maintain fitness levels. A philosophy I like to instill in my clients is, Why lose it when it's so easy to keep?

Research has shown that the effects associated with physical training are indeed transient and reversible if regular training is not possible. On the other hand, recent studies have made it clear that a few days of rest, or a *reduction* in training, will not negatively affect the training process and performance—and may even enhance it. This is especially true for highly trained athletes and is probably related to the importance of recovery in optimizing the adaptation response and avoiding overtraining.

Maintaining Cardiovascular Fitness

The heart is like other muscles in the body. If it is not conditioned by large-muscle, rhythmic activity that simultaneously increases heart rate and a large volume of blood back to the heart, it becomes deconditioned and less efficient at delivering blood and oxygen. A lack of endurance training on a regular basis can significantly compromise the cardiovascular system.

One study showed that after 21 days of complete bed rest, untrained subjects experienced a smaller decrease in $\dot{V}O_2$ max than trained subjects, and regained their initial fitness levels in less time. In fact, it took only 10 days of reconditioning for the untrained subjects to return to their previous fitness levels, versus 40 days for the trained subjects. This demonstrates that a highly trained athlete (or dedicated fitness enthusiast) has more to lose in terms of fitness and takes significantly longer to regain peak performance/conditioning levels.

This observation has important implications for sport conditioning specificity if you compete to win. You need a year-round, periodized training program that includes maintenance phases so that significant levels of fitness are not lost.

The heart strengthens itself in proportion to the force it must contract against. Because of this, periods of inactivity lead to substantial cardiovascular deconditioning. But, even *limited* activity (note that the study mentioned in the previous paragraph used complete bed rest) provides considerable conditioning for the heart. Day-to-day activity provides some maintenance of key cardiovascular functions because the heart must contract forcefully enough to circulate the blood against the demands of gravity. There is a significant difference between complete inactivity (bed rest) and cessation of training because of travel or sickness while one is still participating in normal daily routines.

> **KEY POINT**
>
> Minimal activity—whether it is in the form of a formal workout or simply being busy with daily routine—is an important contribution to maintenance of fitness gains.

Minimal Quantities of Cardiovascular Exercise

Following are the optimal frequency, duration, and level of exercise intensity required to maintain aerobic improvements attained through training.

Early studies found that cardiovascular fitness was maintained by exercising three times per week. Significant losses in endurance conditioning were observed in subjects when they exercised only once or twice per week. Duration and intensity were held constant.

When Less Can Be Enough

Many athletes and fitness enthusiasts would be better off using less time and more effort. This idea is supported by Dr. Robert Hickson, who completed a series of three studies (indirectly referred to on page 240) that led him to a conclusion that "Individuals who have reached a pretty good level of fitness can maintain their fitness fairly easily" (Ken McAlpine, "The Minimalist's Maxim," *Outside Magazine*, April 1993, pg. 163).

The argument for less is relevant to both health-oriented clients and athletes with regard to (1) increased performance, (2) the same or possibly less time commitment, (3) a reduced risk of injury from overtraining, and (4) less chance of personal burnout. You may be training as hard (read this "quantity") as ever and notice that fitness gains, or performance, are falling off. Of course, as you become more fit, fitness gains are harder to come by. But at some point you may wonder, Why keep working so much if it's not doing me any good and isn't that fun?

Many top-ranked athletes and their coaches are putting this thought into action and drastically cutting back on time spent training. Guess what? Training results can improve drastically. Some initial gains might be attributed to rest and recovery, which allow for positive training adaptations to take place in response to the hard efforts. However, what kept the gains coming was another secret ingredient—intensity of effort!

You can maintain any level of fitness with reduced duration and frequency if intensity is maintained. The key is to first attain an acceptable level of fitness. After this, you can worry about maintaining it and manipulating the variables of frequency, intensity, and duration to best fit into your schedule.

Probably the key variable that was identified in more recent research, in regard to a maintenance effect on cardiovascular fitness, was the degree of effort, or intensity. In a landmark study, a reduction in intensity of as little as one-third resulted in significant decreases in $\dot{V}O_2$ max.

KEY POINT

Intensity of training is the primary factor in maintaining the trained state. To maintain cardiovascular fitness, as measured by $\dot{V}O_2$ max (the highest amount of oxygen you can take in and make ATP—energy—aerobically), generally requires at least three training sessions per week at a training intensity of at least 70 percent of $\dot{V}O_2$ max or HRR.

Health or Performance?

The results of these studies should not be interpreted to mean that ex-ercise performed less than three times per week at less than 70 percent of HRR is not valuable. Health gains can be realized with much less exercise and lower intensities. Furthermore, health gains do not necessarily require an increase in $\dot{V}O_2$ max. Other variables can contribute to, for example, increased cardio-vascular endurance, weight loss, and decreased risk for heart disease. Indi-vidual goals and initial fitness levels must be considered.

This information can easily be applied to your current fitness status. Everyone has a percentage of $\dot{V}O_2$ max that corresponds to a steady rate (easy pace) or lower, at which they can easily exercise. A deconditioned person may barely sustain a 2- to 3-mph (30 to 20 minutes per mile) walk. A highly conditioned individual may be able to sustain a 10-mph (six minutes per mile) running pace. Regardless of the fitness level, if either of these specific intensi-ties is reduced by about one-third or greater, a decrease in aerobic conditioning will occur.

However, if intensity is kept constant and no more than a two-thirds reduction in frequency and duration occurs, any physiologic adaptations or health and fitness gains realized will probably be maintained. Put another way, if previous exercise intensity is maintained during a period of lesser training, regardless of your absolute fitness level, the frequency (how often) and duration (how much) of physical activity required to maintain this specific level of aerobic fitness is *less* than that required to improve it.

If you're vacationing, recreating, or on business travel for around 10 days and you're normally active or involved in some type of training on a regular basis, a decrease in structured activity will have little impact on overall health and fitness. It is very encouraging to know that most of your cardiovascular training benefits can be kept by maintaining your current level of effort while simultaneously reducing frequency and duration of effort by as much as two-thirds.

Journalist Ken McAlpine calls it "Training's corollary of compromise: Less is *not* more, but less is often enough! Sometimes you have to give up what you know for what works" (*Outside Magazine*, April 1993). Remember, until you actually get into great shape, you won't get far thinking about minimums, and if you focus on intensity before proper increases in duration and frequency, you risk a greater chance of injury and noncompliance.

Maintaining Muscular Endurance, Strength, and Power

If you're following a regular strength-conditioning program of three sessions a week and miss a workout or so, does your strength greatly decline? Or, if you temporarily cut down on the number of workouts per week, is the result going to be disastrous? Most people have an innate fear that muscular strength and endurance gained through training will be lost after a brief period of time off from their regular training effort. Not to worry, say most researchers! Compared to cardiovascular conditioning, strength is kept over a much longer period of time after detraining begins.

KEY POINT

While levels of strength, power, and muscular endurance are reduced once you stop training, these changes are relatively small during the first few months following the cessation of training.

A few days of recovery or missed workouts will probably have little effect. A week or two of complete inactivity starts to impact these systems, with anaerobic (strength) performance being much easier to maintain.

Development of muscular strength requires an anaerobic effort, and research has shown that maintenance of strength levels requires a fairly small time investment compared to that required to maintain aerobic or muscular endurance capacity.

When an individual breaks an arm or a leg and the broken limb is placed in a rigid cast to immobilize it, changes immediately start taking place in both the bone and surrounding muscles. We now know that skeletal muscles will undergo substantial decreases in size (atrophy) with complete inactivity. Accompanying this decrease in size is a considerable loss in strength and power.

The physiologic mechanisms responsible for this decline in muscle strength with immobilization are not clearly understood. One thought is that muscle disuse also reduces the frequency of neurological stimulation and normal pathways for the recruitment of muscle. Part of the strength loss associated with detraining may result from an inability to activate previously active muscle.

While total inactivity will lead to very rapid losses in both strength and power, periods of *reduced* activity may lead to gradual losses that become significant only as the changes accumulate over long periods of time. Just as in cardiovascular conditioning, being active with daily tasks and reducing training has much less impact on muscle and bone loss than being confined to a bed or immobilized by a cast.

Noted physiologist Dr. David Costill reported that muscle strength and power gained during training can be kept for up to six weeks of *inactivity* (*Sports Medicine Digest*, May 1988). In addition, Costill stated that about 50 percent of the strength gained with training can be maintained for up to a year following the end of the training program. Other studies have shown that it takes less effort to regain lost strength than it does to gain it (*Physician and Sportsmedicine*, 1985). This is welcome news for any athlete who's training schedule is interrupted by life's events.

More exciting than facing the proposition of regaining strength is the fact that research appears to confirm that *maintenance* of strength gains can be prolonged for at least 12 to 16 weeks with minimal stimulation. It appears that intensity rather than exercise duration is the key stimulus for increases in strength. Single-set training seems to be as effective as multiple-set training.

> ## KEY POINT
>
> By working out once every 10 to 14 days, you can maintain the strength, power, and muscular endurance that you gained through more frequent and longer resistance training sessions, if you maintain *intensity* (*Sports Medicine Digest*, May 1988).

When reducing the number of workouts, for example, from three times to once or twice per week, strength can be maintained. Researcher Dr. Graves explains, "If you want to maintain your strength when you are working out less often, you must make sure that your workout is just as difficult as the workout you conduct when you are training more frequently" (Reported in *IDEA Today*, July-August 1989, pg. 13).

Evidently, a muscle requires only a minimal stimulus to retain its strength, power, and size. This has exciting implications if you're injured, and can be a powerful motivator if you have attained a muscular strength and endurance level you would like to maintain but can no longer invest the same time that was necessary to achieve this fitness level.

Maintaining Flexibility Gains

Even though flexibility is gained quickly, it is lost rather quickly during inactivity. Keep flexibility training at the forefront of your program. It is as important as cardiovascular and strength training. While flexibility can be attained in a relatively short period of time, it is in your best interest to maintain functional levels of flexibility on a consistent basis. Reduced flexibility may leave you more susceptible to injury and can affect your actual performance and enjoyment of physical activity. Besides all of this, it feels good!

REGAINING FITNESS

Many studies support the idea that regaining previous fitness levels requires far less effort than it took to first acquire them. This is motivating news, and though I am not in dispute with this thought, I contend that it is far easier to *maintain* some semblance of training and general activity. When you yo-yo between low and high levels of fitness, you risk lack of compliance to your exercise program and possible injury.

It is very disheartening, to say the least, to attain a new level of fitness and health and, for various reasons, lose a majority of the gained benefits. As life straightens out, you will resolve once again to get on the perfect program. Do yourself a favor and realize that no such beast exists. These situations often occur because many people have been set up with a philosophy of all or none in terms of their approach to an exercise program, and life in general. This learned attitude emboldens the philosophy that if you cannot embrace the training regime with optimal time investment and consistency, why do it at all? This is the perfection scheme that sets many exercisers up for personal failure with regard to their exercise and nutrition programs. With the research presented previously, it is obvious that some of something is better than nothing. Consistency and moderation are in, and they work! This reasonable approach is effective and supported by research. Also, it is quite easy to maintain, or regain, fitness levels with smart and sensible training.

If you stop exercising for two weeks or longer, do not pick up where you left off. Start at a lower intensity, for instance, less resistance, slower speeds, and shorter durations. The odds are that you will regain your previous levels of fitness fairly quickly if you allow for this progressive adaptation to the new stresses you are placing on your body. Temper your enthusiasm and desire to start out too intensely.

Missing an exercise session periodically will not greatly affect current levels of fitness. Regardless of your fitness level and component of fitness being trained, intensity of effort is the key factor to optimizing training effects and creating results-oriented use of time. Reducing training frequency and duration will not drastically affect fitness as long as training intensity is maintained. Remember, doing something is far superior to doing nothing.

TAKING YOUR FITNESS TO THE NEXT LEVEL

Results start with a dream, an idea, and a time commitment to your vision. The successful path continues with a growing knowledge base and accurate information. Your program goes nowhere without a goal-oriented plan of action and an objective evaluative process that tells you whether your program is working.

Reevaluating Your Goals

Would you like your fitness program to push on toward the standards of personal health and fitness you have set? Revisit your goals, both long- and short-term, and keep track of your efforts. Evaluate your progress by reassessing your fitness level regularly and graphing your progress on the performance graph. The information that you accumulate or read about is useful to you only if you *use* it! Put the programs in this book to work. Take action and follow through so you will have a complete approach to designing and monitoring your fitness program to ensure maximum results.

The evaluation and testing sheets, performance graphs, and workout record-keeping logs provided in this book will make it easy for you to keep a written record of your program. It is from this objective information, recorded when your memory is sharp and accurate, that you can get a true sense of whether your program is performance- and results-oriented and progressing. Compare your workout progress to your current goals. Are they in line with one another, or do you need to make a change? Remember, it takes time, consistent effort, and accurate record keeping to stay on track with your workouts and to attain your goals.

> ### KEY POINT
>
> Reassess your current goals and set new goals to keep your program fresh, producing results, and realistic.

Monitoring your training efforts and setting new goals are exciting processes because they demonstrate the results you are getting from your dedicated and planned efforts. Results don't just happen. They occur because you have put in conscientious thought and preplanned your route, and you have carried out the orders! A successful direction is impossible without first setting goals and following these with updated versions that reflect your current situation.

Adjusting Your Workouts

More programs fail, not because an individual doesn't know what to do, but because the person fails to act on the knowledge he or she already possesses. Change is good. Take charge and move forward. Use your self-test results and record-keeping sheets to determine the effectiveness of your programs. Set goals to elevate your motivation and desire.

Your Personal Trainer provides the right tools and accurate information so that you can continue to move your fitness to new levels. The combination of self-testing/assessment, interval training, strength training, fueling your workouts with the right food, cross-training, periodizing your workout program, and having easy-to-use tracking/record-keeping forms are the essentials you need to move your program to optimal heights. This book was meant to use. So, here's to you in good health and performance...now get busy!

Quick Index:

Appendix

RESOURCES

Equipment

Elastic resistance and tubing

Lifeline International, Inc., 800-553-6633; fax: 608-288-9294;

SPRI, Inc., 800-222-7774; fax: 847-537-4941;

and SIL, Inc., 800-824-9652; fax: 908-206-1809.

Three excellent companies that supply elastic resistance training systems, assorted tubing and other fitness products like exercise mats. Call or fax for a free catalog or to order.

Magnetic microload weight add-on

PlateMates: SIL, Inc., 800-824-9652; fax: 908-206-1809, for information or to order.

Multi-station strength training gym

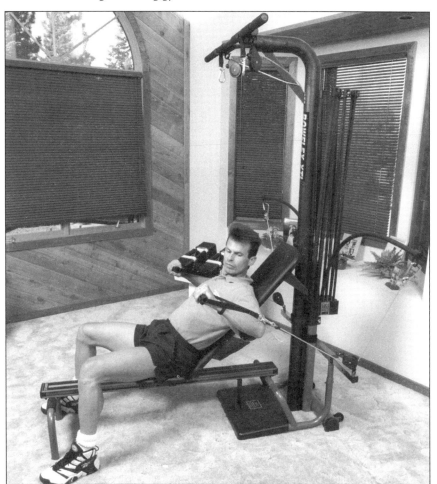

Bowflex Strength Training Systems, 800-819-3539, 360-694-7722; fax: 360-694-7755, to request a free brochure, video tape or to order. (Basic unit, suggested retail, $1,000.00)

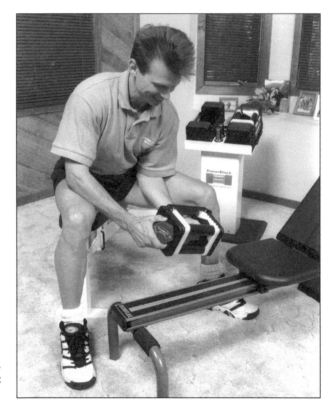

Selectorized dumbbells

> PowerBlock Dumbbell System: Intell Bell, Inc., 800-446-5215, 507-451-5152; fax: 507-451-5278

Skinfold caliper

> Accu-Measure, Inc., P.O. Box 4040, Parker Colorado 80134, USA. 800-866-2727; fax 303-690-4219 (Suggested retail, $19.95)

Stability ball

> Air-filled exercise ball. Moves International, 800-272-5055, 760-934-0312; fax: 760-934-2535; email: movesint@qnet.com

> The supplier of stability balls and stability ball instructional manuals and videos, as well as numerous strength, stretch, and step videos.

Nutritional Software

> Diet Balancer. 800-927-2988.

> DINE Healthy.
> Dine Systems Inc. 800-688-1848

> Nutri-Calc.
> Cande Corporation. 602-926-2632

Reading Material

> Clark, Nancy. 1997. *Nancy Clark's Sports Nutrition Guidebook: Eating to Fuel Your Active Lifestyle.* Champaign, IL: Human Kinetics Publishers (800-747-4457).

> If you want more information on sports nutrition, this is the only book you'll need.

Index

About the Author

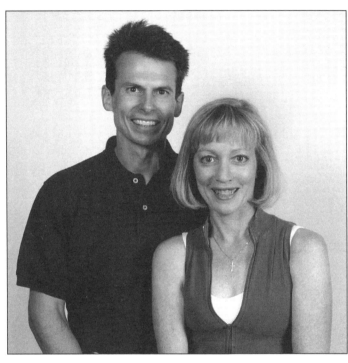

Known as the "trainer's trainer," Douglas Brooks is one of the premier personal trainers in the United States. He's widely recognized through his numerous appearances on home shopping networks, infomercials, the Cable Health Club Network, and fitness videos. An ACE-certified personal trainer since 1983, Brooks is also the fitness training director at Snowcreek Resort and Athletic Club and the co-owner of Moves International, a provider of educational resources, continuing education, and live workshops for fitness professionals.

Brooks has also authored *Going Solo: The Art of Personal Training*—a landmark publication written during personal training's infancy—and *Program Design for Personal Trainers: Bridging Theory Into Application,* as well as numerous educational manuals. He is active in many professional organizations, including IDEA—The Health and Fitness Source, the International Sports Trainers Association, the American College of Sports Medicine, and the National Strength and Conditioning Association. He also conducts lectures and workshops throughout the United States and internationally on the topics of personal training, strength training, kinesiology, and exercise physiology.

Brooks enjoys fitness activities of all kinds. He is a competitive tennis player, marathoner, Ironman triathlete, alpine and nordic skier, in-line skater, rock climber, and mountaineer. He holds a master's degree in exercise physiology from Central Michigan University. Brooks, his wife, Candice, and their two sons live in Mammoth Lakes, California.

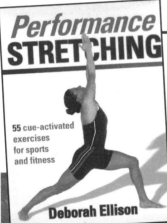
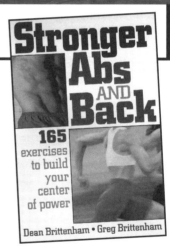
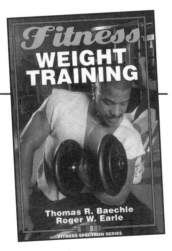